DATE DUE

GAYLORD			PRINTED IN U.S.A.

UNDERMINING SCIENCE

Undermining Science

Suppression and Distortion
in the Bush Administration

Seth Shulman

UNIVERSITY OF CALIFORNIA PRESS Berkeley Los Angeles London

University of California Press, one of the most distinguished university presses in the United States, enriches
lives around the world by advancing scholarship in the
humanities, social sciences, and natural sciences. Its activities are supported by the UC Press Foundation and
by philanthropic contributions from individuals and institutions. For more information, visit
www.ucpress.edu.

University of California Press
Berkeley and Los Angeles, California

University of California Press, Ltd.
London, England

Library of Congress Cataloging-in-Publication Data

Shulman. Seth.
    Undermining science : suppression and distortion in
the Bush Administration / Seth Shulman.
        p. cm.
    Includes bibliographical references and index.
    ISBN-13: 978-0-520-24702-4 (cloth : alk. paper)
    ISBN-10: 0-520-24702-7 (cloth : alk. paper)
    1. Science and state—United States.   2. Research—
Political aspects—United States.   3. United States—
Political and government—2001–   4. Pressure groups.
I. Title.

Q127.U6S58   2007
509.73'090511—dc22   2006017924

Manufactured in the United States of America

15   14   13   12   11   10   09   08   07   06
10   9   8   7   6   5   4   3   2   1

The paper used in this publication meets the minimum
requirements of ANSI/NISO Z39.48-1992 (R 1997) (Per-
manence of Paper).

for Laura,
explorer, partner, muse

It is increasingly impossible to ignore that this White House disdains research that inconveniences it.

Editorial, *Scientific American*, May 2004

Contents

Preface

On February 18, 2004, more than sixty of the most eminent scientists in the United States gave an unprecedented vote of no confidence to the administration of George W. Bush. The scientists who came forward, including Nobel laureates, National Medal of Science recipients, and members of the National Academy of Sciences, had all signed a statement, entitled *Restoring Scientific Integrity in Policy Making,* which charged the administration with a widespread pattern of suppression and distortion across numerous federal agencies.

With the 2004 presidential election approaching, the nation was highly polarized at the time of the announcement, yet the scientists' statement could not be easily written off as a partisan attack. The signatories were too distinguished and diverse to ignore. Some, like Paul Berg, Harold Varmus, and Herbert York, had opened vast new horizons in genetic engineering, medicine, and military technology. Others, like Lewis Branscomb, Neal Lane, and Russell Train, had served as prominent advisers to Democratic and Republican presidents.

To raise the public ire of this group, something had to be seriously wrong.

After all, science depends upon impartiality and independent thinking; scientists rarely issue group statements, particularly in such numbers and on sweeping issues. As the saying goes, you might as well try to herd cats as to get a group of prominent scientists to agree to a joint state-ment—especially an overtly *political* statement. As much as they eschew group pronouncements, most scientists also tend to avoid the political fray. To be sure, individual scientists often weigh in with expert testi-mony on specific matters of science policy or engage in political affairs in their private lives. But their professional work teaches them to draw narrow conclusions from their research. Scientists' analytic training, as well as the culture of the enterprise, reinforces the notion that they should avoid overgeneralization at all cost.

Yet here they were, in February 2004, declaring that:

> When scientific knowledge has been found to be in conflict with its polit-ical goals, the administration has often manipulated the process through which science enters into its decisions. This has been done by placing people who are professionally unqualified or who have clear conflicts of interest in official posts and on scientific advisory committees; by dis-banding existing advisory committees; by censoring and suppressing re-ports by the government's own scientists; and by simply not seeking inde-pendent scientific advice. Other administrations have, on occasion, engaged in such practices, but not so systematically nor on so wide a front. Furthermore, in advocating policies that are not scientifically sound, the administration has sometimes misrepresented scientific knowledge and misled the public about the implications of its policies.[1]

What had galvanized these scientists into action?

The answer is quite straightforward. Facts. Scientists recognize that they cannot do their jobs—that the entire scientific enterprise will col-lapse—if they do not faithfully record and report their data. Whenever scientists suppress findings or, worse, cook their books, not only do they set their fields back terribly, they jeopardize their colleagues, whose work necessarily builds upon that of others. Not surprisingly, when the perpetrators of such infractions are discovered, they are normally drummed out of the profession. Clearly, these prominent U.S. scientists found themselves unable to overlook a disturbing and unacceptable reality: the federal administration of George W. Bush was systematically suppressing and manipulating the scientific findings of government sci-entists.

Of course, there are always political considerations in government de-liberations about science policy, but the scientists felt they needed to draw a line. For them, the issues were clear: you don't manipulate the process for collecting scientific information, and you don't suppress scientific data just because it doesn't agree with your political views.

I began collecting the case studies in this book in preparation for writing the detailed report upon which the scientists' statement in February 2004 was based. I did so at the behest of the Union of Concerned Scientists (UCS), an advocacy group that lives up to its name. They believed something was going badly awry in the handling of scientific and technical information in the administration of George W. Bush, and they were more than a little, well, *concerned* about it. I first met with members of the group in 2003. As a roomful of scientists and policy analysts explained to me at that meeting, reports coming in from across the federal government indicated an unprecedented level of political interference and manipulation in the collecting, processing, and release of scientific information and data. Ideologues with dubious credentials were replacing top-notch scientists on advisory panels. Some government scientists were reporting that their work was being censored or even distorted.

By the summer of 2003, at conferences and in labs around the country, many scientists had begun talking with one another about the situation. In Congress, the minority staff of the House Committee on Government Reform, under the auspices of Rep. Henry Waxman (D-CA), had issued a report on the matter that had begun to circulate widely.

The Union of Concerned Scientists felt that it ought to do something about the issue but was unsure how best to address the subject. The group was highly effective in analyzing the technical aspects of science policy. Its members had published and testified widely about issues ranging from global warming to ballistic missile defense. But this was different. The issue was extremely broad, involving the mechanics of how the government conducted science. And addressing that subject head-on required just the kind of overtly political and seemingly partisan discourse that makes scientists uncomfortable. As a result, the group had contacted me—an independent investigative journalist specializing in science and technology—in the hope that I would look into the matter.

This was new terrain for both sides. For their part, the scientists had grave doubts about wading into this political morass and wondered how they might possibly build a credible investigation out of what was, at the time, a loose patchwork of anecdotes. They didn't know how to substantiate the allegations being levied from many quarters about the Bush administration, and they didn't want to engage in partisan mudslinging. In keeping with the basic tenet of scientific inquiry, they felt the first step was an independent assessment of the evidence.

For my part, while I had done a variety of contract work as a writer and editor, the prospect of working as a journalist for an advocacy group raised some professional questions. Could I retain my independence? Would I compromise my journalistic credibility if I spoke with governmental officials as working on a "Union of Concerned Scientists" project?

I had other doubts as well. As I explained during the first meeting, I was worried that the problem was difficult to communicate to the public. Many people hold the cynical—and not unreasonable—view that politics have always pervaded science policy. To them, the whole thing might seem like nothing more than a bunch of elitist scientists whining that the current administration was ignoring them.

After some deliberation, we agreed that I would undertake a preliminary investigation. I would be free to pursue the issue in any way I saw fit and to use the information I gathered in any way I chose. Based on my findings, however, I would write a private memo for the Union of Concerned Scientists that assessed the allegations that had begun to surface about the lack of scientific integrity in the Bush administration.

None of us in the fall of 2003 had any inkling of the extent and pervasiveness of politicization that I would encounter. As skeptical as I might have been at the outset, once I began to speak to government scientists at numerous federal agencies, I soon had little doubt that the administration was involved in a concerted campaign to deceive the American public on a breathtaking array of issues.

This book, based on scores of interviews with officials inside and outside the federal government through the summer of 2005, documents how the Bush administration lost the confidence of the scientific community through selective suppression and distortion of the research of government scientists and policy analysts. Taken together, the stories presented here expose a calculated strategy by the administration to mislead the public about research conducted at dozens of federal agencies on vital issues of public health, environmental degradation, and national security. As I will document, in many separate realms the administration has repeatedly allowed partisan political considerations to corrupt the integrity of the government's role as a broker of scientific information and assessment. The degree of lying, deception, and manipulation of information reported across so many federal agencies would seem to have required in the administration of George W. Bush a combination of callousness, mendacity, and hubris that is rare even in the messy history of American politics.

For the past several years, this story has come to dominate my professional life. Not only did the Union of Concerned Scientists publish the initial findings in a widely read report in February 2004, my follow-up report for the organization was released in July of that year, and I have continued to document the administration's mishandling of scientific information since then.

To date, in an effort coordinated by the Union of Concerned Scientists, more than eight thousand U.S. scientists have signed the statement originally released in February 2004. As of the spring of 2006, the signers included some 49 Nobel laureates, 63 National Medal of Science recipients, and 171 members of the National Academy of Sciences. The effort has generated thousands of news stories around the world and garnered widespread television and radio coverage. Two editorials in the *New York Times*, for example, explicitly endorsed the findings of the initial UCS report.[2] Even more notably, the scientists' charges—along with similar accusations from many quarters—have come to define a now-well-accepted hallmark of the Bush administration: as a front-page headline in the *Washington Post* put it as early as October 2002: "For Bush, Facts Are Malleable."[3]

More recently, a barrage of incidents—from the federal response to Hurricane Katrina to Bush administration policies on torture and domestic wiretapping—have led a majority of Americans to believe that the administration routinely misleads the public, and not just on science, according to recent polls.[4] The incidents documented here were among the first to draw this issue to public attention and to publicly define this modus operandi of the administration.

When the Union of Concerned Scientists' report was released in February 2004, the first-term Bush administration, presumably recognizing the seriousness of the scientists' charges in an election year, issued a point-by-point rebuttal. The White House Office of Science and Technology Policy released a 14-page statement by U.S. science adviser John H. Marburger III, claiming that the descriptions of the incidents in the report were all "false," "wrong," or "misleading."[5] But when a team of scientists and staffers at the Union of Concerned Scientists reviewed the particulars cited in Marburger's response, it could publicly document that in virtually every instance his explanations were either irrelevant to the cases presented or insufficient to explain them away. The Union of Concerned Scientists, after subjecting its report to the closest scrutiny from experts inside and outside the organization, ultimately stood by the initial document in its entirety.[6]

Since that official exchange—well before the 2004 presidential election—the Bush administration has been virtually silent on the issue. The scientists may have had their facts straight, but, as it turned out, their accuracy won them only a Pyrrhic victory. Despite the public attention the efforts of the Union of Concerned Scientists received, other factors overshadowed the lapses in scientific integrity documented in the reports. Fear of terrorism and the wars in Afghanistan and Iraq dominated the public's attention; George W. Bush narrowly won a second term in office. Meanwhile, the suppression and manipulation of scientific information has continued apace.

Sadly, as I will show in detail, during George W. Bush's tenure, a new standard has been set for the overt politicization of government efforts to collect and disseminate information, significantly eroding the credibility of Washington—and not just in matters of science and technology. It is a disturbing trend and one that is not easily rectified. And despite what some cynics might say, it is not politics as usual; it is something more serious. As the expression goes, reputations are built slowly but damaged quickly. The reputation of the U.S. government as a fair broker of scientific information has been badly damaged. Rebuilding it will require perseverance, care, and honesty; many career government scientists have left the public sector in disgust, and many more are deeply demoralized by the overt politicization of their work and the unprecedented levels of ideologically based censorship and micromanagement in which they must now operate.

Nonetheless, the historical pendulum swings; democratic societies frequently demonstrate the capacity to learn from the mistakes of one set of elected officials and to take corrective action in legislation and new leadership. I am confident that the American public will eventually take such corrective action on this matter.

In fact, when Reed Malcolm, an editor at the University of California Press, suggested that I write a book on this topic, I accepted in part because I believe these stories have not just current but historical significance. After all, students still study the infamous cronyism of Boss Tweed and Tammany Hall in the 1860s and 1870s. They study the misguided politicization of science led by the Stalin-era geneticist Trofim Lysenko in the 1930s. They study the zealous anti-communism of U.S. senator Joseph McCarthy in the 1950s, as well as other examples of historical hubris and folly. Perhaps the episodes recounted here will similarly serve as cautionary tales about the importance of honesty and transparency in government and about how easily both can be undermined.

Quite frankly, I also welcomed the chance to write this book because, after a great deal of relatively restrained and decorous reporting for the Union of Concerned Scientists, I wanted to underscore the issues at stake in more explicit and personal language: any fair-minded reader should be able to see that, in the Bush administration, government officials have repeatedly lied to the American public as part of a strategy to further ideological and partisan political ends. As the Latin expression goes, *res ipsa loquitur*—the facts speak for themselves.

Those who signed the Union of Concerned Scientists statement felt compelled to speak out about the manipulation of scientific information. Similarly, as a working journalist, I feel compelled to speak out when the government systematically lies to its citizenry. Too often, in the name of "balance," journalists shy away from declaring explicitly that government officials are lying, preferring to pit the claims of a source on one side of the political aisle against those of another one across the way. Such a reportorial strategy can work effectively only when both sides are mustering evidence to fairly debate a policy issue. Democracy depends upon debate of conflicting views and interests, but that debate can only be meaningful when it rests on truth and honesty. That is not the case in Washington in the era of George W. Bush.

While all such characterizations are mine and mine alone, nonetheless, the detailed case studies presented here owe an enormous debt to the work of many talented people. Perhaps most of all, I want to thank the scores of government scientists, science advisors, and other officials who have spoken out about these issues, including Andrew Eller, Michael Kelly, Bruce Buckheit, Rick Piltz, Gerald Keusch, Bruce Lanphear, Michael Weitzman, Russell Train, and Neal Lane—and many, many more who offered me information but withheld their names for fear of retribution in their current government positions. This book could not have been written without their courageous testimony.

At the Union of Concerned Scientists, Suzanne Shaw offered invaluable editorial and reportorial guidance. Kurt Gottfried, an eminent scientist, provided tremendous energy and helpful input on many of the findings presented here. Many others at UCS and elsewhere offered editorial, technical, or legal help, including close review of portions of the reports the organization produced. For that painstaking work, I thank Michael Bean, Morrow Cater, Nancy Cole, Peter Frumhoff, David Grimes, Lisbeth Gronlund, Kevin Knobloch, Arielle Lutwick, Michelle Manion, Margaret Mellon, Alden Meyer, Kirsten Moore, Joan Mulhern, Gordon Orians, Anthony Robbins, Lexi Shultz, James Trussell, and Bryan Wadsworth.

For their pioneering and continuing work on this subject I am indebted to Josh Sharfstein, Naomi Seiler, and other members, past and present, of the minority staff at the U.S. House Committee on Government Reform. Under the direction of Rep. Henry Waxman, they have worked unflaggingly to try to make this administration accountable for its actions. I am grateful too, as all Americans should be, for the outstanding work of journalists who have reported extensively on many of the cases I describe: Andrew Revkin of the *New York Times,* Tom Hamburger of the *Los Angeles Times,* Rick Weiss of the *Washington Post,* and the freelance writer Chris C. Mooney—as well as many others whose reporting is cited among this book's notes.

Finally, on a more personal note, I want to thank my agent, Katinka Matson, for all her efforts on my behalf. I am grateful to Reed Malcolm at the University of California Press for his enthusiasm for this project and to his editorial staff for their constructive comments and the careful editing needed to bring this volume to fruition. I thank my good friend Marc Miller for his extensive efforts to improve my prose, and my father, Roy Shulman, for his unflagging moral support and interest in my work.

Most of all, though, I am grateful beyond words to my wonderful family—Laura, Elise, and Ben—who helped me every step of the way and remained cheerful even on those long days these past few months when work to complete this manuscript often compelled me, reluctantly, to neglect their admittedly more appealing activities.

1

Facts Matter

Science, like any field of endeavor, relies on freedom of inquiry; and one of the hallmarks of that freedom is objectivity. Now more than ever, on issues ranging from climate change to AIDS research to genetic engineering to food additives, government relies on the impartial perspective of science for guidance.

PRESIDENT GEORGE H. W. BUSH, 1990

The U.S. government runs on information—vast amounts of it. Researchers at the National Weather Service gather and analyze meteorological data so they know when to issue severe-weather advisories. Specialists at the Federal Reserve Bank collect and analyze economic data to determine when to raise or lower interest rates. Experts at the Centers for Disease Control examine bacteria and viral samples to help guard against a large-scale outbreak of disease. The public relies upon the accuracy of such data and upon the integrity of the researchers who gather and analyze it.

Equally important, the analysis of fact-based data is pivotal to the government's policymaking process. When compelling evidence suggests a threat to human health from the presence of minuscule amounts of a contaminant in the water supply, the federal government may move to tighten drinking water standards to protect the public. When data indicate structural problems in aging bridges in the interstate highway system, the federal government may move to allocate emergency repair funds. When the population of an animal species perilously declines, officials may opt to list it for protection under the Endangered Species Act.

Given the myriad pressing problems involving complex scientific and technological data—from the AIDS pandemic to the threat of nuclear proliferation—the public expects government experts and researchers to provide a high caliber of data and analysis, perhaps higher than ever before. One might imagine that impartial researchers with expertise in gathering and analyzing specialized data would be prized for the important role they play in laying the foundation for an informed policymaking process.

And yet the administration of George W. Bush has badly undermined this cornerstone of fact-based data. Scientists, policymakers, and technical specialists affiliated with nearly every federal agency have documented in detail the ways in which Bush administration officials, determined to push through particular political agendas, have systematically ignored, suppressed, or distorted the information gathered and analyzed on their behalf by federal agencies and advisory panels.

As this book will demonstrate, top administration officials have rewritten the work of government scientists on climate change. They have fired leading experts on scientific advisory panels and replaced them with ideologues whose credentials are often questionable at best. And they have routinely tried to shelve government reports whose findings conflict with administration policies.

Politics always plays a central role in science and technology policymaking. Every administration is influenced to some degree by political considerations on matters of science and technology—as it should be. What distinguishes the Bush administration, however, is a dramatic shift: its willingness to stifle or distort scientific evidence from its own federal agencies that runs counter to its preferred policies—and ideologies.

This is a troubling development, unprecedented in both scope and pervasiveness. At the highest levels, the Bush administration has allowed partisan considerations and the influence of special interests to permeate the traditionally nonpartisan mechanisms through which the government gathers, analyzes, and disseminates information. Reasonable people may well disagree over many of the Bush administration's political choices. There is, however, a crucial difference between disputes over policy and the manipulation of the policymaking process itself. Partisanship aside, there should be little disagreement about the need for credibility in the governmental policymaking process.

To understand this distinction, it is important to recognize the difference between policymaking and the practice of scientific assessment and analysis.

Policymaking is about making choices, often difficult ones. How much of a given contaminant should be allowed in drinking water? Should the government require seat belts in automobiles? Should it invest in a new weapon system? To make policy choices, government officials frequently must balance the needs of one constituency against another—a process that embodies the very definition of "politics" itself. Proposed regulations to improve worker safety and health, for example, need to be weighed against the potential economic burden they might place upon small business owners. Tighter auto emissions standards must be considered against the added production costs they will impose upon the auto industry and, in turn, upon consumers if it means higher vehicle prices.

Scientific assessment and technical analysis are quite a different matter. These practices are about finding the best answers we can to specific questions about phenomena and causality in the world. They are, in other words, about identifying and understanding facts as accurately as possible. Scientific information and technical analysis thus provide the underpinning of the policymaking process. Most governmental policymakers understand the crucial importance of robust and impartial sources of information. Put simply, good decision makers seek the best facts they can get. The business of scientists and policy analysts is to try to provide decision makers with that crucial foundation.

It is worth noting that critics, on both the left and right of the political spectrum, often make astute points about the inherent biases that can taint scientific research. Conservatives frequently belittle governmental and academic scientists for essentially being too detached from reality: conducting esoteric studies with taxpayer funds and using the trappings of science and inductive reasoning to hide a liberal bias. Critics on the left, meanwhile, tend to emphasize the extent to which scientists, like everyone else, are enmeshed and influenced by their own political and financial ties. As Richard Lewontin asked in an article on the subject in the *New York Review of Books:* "Why should we trust scientists, who, after all, have their own political and economic agendas?"[1]

Notwithstanding the validity of such critiques, they are largely irrelevant to the case studies of outright distortion and censorship presented here. Clearly, governmental scientists and technical analysts are not infallibly objective or unbiased. But the degree to which bias taints these practitioners—whether they are "too aloof in their liberal beliefs" or "too entrenched in the elite establishment"—fades to background noise if an entire policymaking system is consciously manipulated for partisan gain. Discussing such issues, given the extraordinary circumstances reported by government scientists and technical analysts working in the Bush administration, is rather like conducting an argument about the extent to which pilots normally deviate from their flight plan while riding in an airplane that has just been hijacked.

AN UNPRECEDENTED POLITICIZATION

Consider one small but telling incident. In November 2003, a National Cancer Institute fact sheet was altered, over government scientists' objections, to lend credence to a favorite canard of some anti-abortion Christian conservatives that there is a link between abortion and breast cancer. A number of scientific studies—most notably a highly respected Danish study in the 1990s involving *1.5 million* women—have thoroughly refuted the link.[2] And yet, as has frequently occurred in the Bush administration, politics—whether out of ideological conviction or to appease political partisans—trumped peer-reviewed scientific evidence, and a federal agency was pushed to dispense misleading information about a vital matter of women's health. After a public outcry, including a *New York Times* editorial labeling the incident "an egregious distortion of the evidence," the National Cancer Institute restored its public information to reflect the well-documented scientific evidence that no connection exists between abortion and breast cancer.[3]

The most notable thing about this incident is that it happened at all. This was not a question of bias or incompetence quietly creeping into the government's dissemination of scientific information; it reflects a wholesale effort to mislead the public on behalf of anti-abortion activists. It is one thing for such groups to peddle misinformation on the World Wide Web and elsewhere about the bogus cancer connection to try to frighten women out of having abortions. It is quite another for the National Cancer Institute to condone the politically motivated manipulation of data.

The issue of whether or not one opposes abortion is a moral and political question. The question of whether a link exists between abortion and breast cancer is *not* a political question. It is an empirical question about the most up-to-date and best-supported scientific knowledge.

In the extraordinary climate created by the Bush administration, though, it is not enough for scientists to investigate the facts of a given situation; they now must often explain to policymakers that facts matter in the first place. As the eminent Stanford University scientist Richard N. Zare wrote in the *San Francisco Chronicle* in 2005, "We must be willing to speak out against the threat of making science just a matter of opinion." "Scientific theories are more than a special set of opinions that the scientific community is trying to push onto the public in opposition to religious beliefs," noted Zare, who served on the National Science Board under presidents Clinton and Bush senior. "To pretend otherwise is to invite the decline of our nation."[4]

To understand more about the current climate, consider the situation of a senior government scientist who has served both Democratic and Republican presidents. Speaking to me after-hours from his home because of fear of retribution, he cited eight instances in which his colleagues were denied the opportunity to present papers, prohibited from submitting their articles to journals, or ordered to significantly alter their findings for a government document or report. In each instance, he said, the actions were taken not because the researchers' work was poorly executed but rather "because the findings were not consistent with administration policies."[5]

"Scientific integrity is being badly impaired," he told me, adding that he had seen nothing like it in nearly twenty years as a government scientist. I corroborated much of his story from other sources, but, alas, was unable to persuade him to allow me to go public with the particulars. The details of his story are so clearly identifiable that, even if I withheld his name, the source of the leak would be obvious. He agonized about the situation but ultimately felt he had to put the welfare of his family first; he could not risk losing his job.

Even so, this source, and many others like him, helped me to understand the climate of fear and demoralization that now pervades scientific work in many federal agencies. This particular scientist, for instance, explained that researchers at his agency are routinely subjected to tight control by the administration. He told me that each technical area in his agency has "political commissars"—all political appointees—whose job is to make sure that scientific and technical work conducted within the government does not conflict with the administration's political agenda.

What makes this source particularly compelling is how fundamentally apolitical he is. He made it clear to me that his complaint lies not with the administration's policy choices but with its profoundly undemocratic processes. As he put it: "All government scientists want the same thing: a fair hearing for their research and a chance to put their data on the table." In the administration of George W. Bush, this chance is being systematically denied.

AN AFFRONT TO SCIENCE AND DEMOCRACY

It is easy enough to understand why the politically motivated censorship and distortion of scientific and technical research would be of overriding concern even to apolitical scientists: a doctrinaire allegiance to one set of conclusions violates the central premise of the scientific method. As the conservative philosopher Karl Popper famously explained in his classic work *The Logic of Scientific Discovery,* science achieves a deeper understanding of the world precisely by vigorously challenging hypotheses, a process Popper dubbed as "falsification." For scientists, Popper wrote, the method of research is not to defend previous findings but "using all the weapons of our logical, mathematical, and technical armory" to "try to overthrow them." As Popper put it, "Those among us who are unwilling to expose their ideas to the hazard of refutation do not take part in the scientific game."[6]

In this context, the reaction within the scientific community to the administration's actions is unsurprising. Pseudoscientific or "faith-based" interventions, in contradiction to observable evidence, are being promoted and funded with taxpayer money, while valuable lifesaving innovations are stifled or neglected. Many researchers now find their work censored by the administration, while others engage in self-censorship as a defense against losing their jobs. Many other scientists and technical specialists have left government service in despair or protest. The Centers for Disease Control have been hit particularly hard. As many as forty top CDC managers—in career positions—have left the agency since the start of the Bush administration, according to the *Washington Post.*[7]

As serious as these effects are for scientists and the scientific community, the impact is even more grave for the health of the nation's democratic processes. Consider, for instance, the assessment in 2004 of Rep. Brian Baird (D-WA), a member of the House Science Committee: "In countless subtle and not so subtle ways," Baird contends, "the administration and Republican majorities who control the House and Senate are deliberately and systematically suppressing discussion and criticism and distorting the scientific process. The modalities of such distortions are manifold and collectively constitute nothing less than a coordinated attack on virtually every stage and aspect of the science/policy interaction."[8]

In a campaign spanning virtually every federal agency, the Bush administration has employed an arsenal of tactics to undermine scientific integrity.

SUBVERTING THE WORK OF GOVERNMENT SCIENTISTS

By vesting unprecedented power in a small cadre of White House loyalists, the administration has censored and distorted the work of agency scientists throughout the government. As detailed in chapter 2, one of the clearest examples of this strategy has been to allow a close-knit group of industry-friendly nonscientists at the White House's Council on Environmental Quality to tightly control all scientific research conducted throughout the federal government on the issue of global warming. The administration has required that virtually every piece of scientific research and assessment on climate change funnel through this small, politically motivated group. In so doing, the White House has subverted the independence of federal agencies by making sure any scientific assessments released by the government conform to predetermined administration policy positions.

SUPPRESSING ANALYSES THAT DIVERGE FROM PREFERRED POLICY

Whether in science or other technical arenas, when dissenting analyses *have* surfaced within the federal government, the administration has frequently squelched them. This happened, for example, in November 2003, just before Congress voted in favor of the administration's massive Medicare reform bill. Richard Foster, the chief actuary for the federal Medicare program, sought to release to Congress his analysis showing that the bill would cost $500 billion to $600 billion over ten years, *as much as $200 billion more* than the White House's official estimate.

Thomas Scully, the administration's Medicare chief, threatened to fire Foster if he released his analysis. As a result, Congress passed a bill that was based on numbers the administration knew to be inaccurate. After the story broke but before Congress could complete its feckless investigation of Scully's behavior, he resigned to work as a lobbyist for the pharmaceutical industry. As an editorial in the *New York Times* lamented after the deception came to light: "it is a terrible policy to deprive legislators of information they need to make informed choices."[9]

INJECTING POLITICS INTO SCIENTIFIC DETERMINATIONS

In many scientific arenas, the Bush administration has made a habit of injecting overtly political considerations into decisions that are normally debated on their scientific merits. As discussed in chapter 4, for example, the Food and Drug Administration (FDA) is required by law to approve drugs that are found to be safe and effective. In an almost unprecedented repudiation of governmental scientific expertise, however, Steven Galson, acting director of the FDA's Center for Drug Evaluation and Research, overturned the recommendations of his own staff and two FDA advisory panels and refused to approve over-the-counter access to the emergency "morning-after" contraceptive pill levonorgestrel, sold under the brand name Plan B.[10]

Although members of the two FDA scientific advisory committees had voted overwhelmingly to recommend over-the-counter access and stated that such a decision would present "no issues" of concern to women's health, the normal process of approval was circumvented.[11] Through the intervention of Dr. David Hager, a highly controversial evangelist physician appointed to the FDA advisory panel, the Bush administration blocked easier access to this contraceptive and pandered to religious activists who oppose birth control.

ALLOWING INDUSTRY AND OTHER INTEREST GROUPS TO INTERFERE IN GOVERNMENTAL PROCESSES

The Bush administration has frequently allowed private industry representatives to intervene in—and even dictate the outcome of—governmental policymaking. For example, as detailed in chapter 5, reports by both the Government Accountability Office (GAO) and the inspector general of the Environmental Protection Agency (EPA) determined that top officials interfered with EPA scientists to suppress and distort analyses of mercury emissions from power plants. As part of this policy-making process, the EPA's proposed rule on mercury emissions contained no fewer than twelve paragraphs lifted, sometimes verbatim, from a legal document prepared by industry lawyers. Chagrined EPA officials explained that the language had crept into the preamble to their proposed rules "through the interagency process."[12] But the example underscores the lack of public input in the process and the tight and often secret circles of influence that operate routinely in the current administration.

STACKING SCIENTIFIC ADVISORY PANELS

The Bush administration has dramatically politicized the process through which appointments are made to science advisory panels. Although the appointment process has always involved political considerations, past administrations have historically looked for some political breadth and great scientific depth. Such considerations have been virtually ignored in the current administration. In one well-documented case in 2002, Tommy Thompson, as secretary of the Department of Health and Human Services, summarily rejected three well-qualified ergonomics experts from a peer review panel at the National Institute for Occupational Safety and Health (NIOSH).[13] The three nominees in question had been selected to join a study section of the Advisory Committee on Occupational Safety and Health that evaluates research grants on workplace injuries.[14] The committee chair and panel staff had chosen the three based on their credentials and reputations in the field, and the director of NIOSH had initially approved the appointments.

What makes this example so noteworthy is that so-called study sections are responsible for conducting peer review of ongoing research, not for advising on policy matters, and therefore changes of administration have almost never affected them. Traditionally, scientists in such positions are chosen strictly for their relevant expertise, just as their peer review work requires them to assess research solely based on its scientific merit. In this case, however, Thompson rejected at least two of the nominees because of their support for a workplace ergonomics standard, a policy opposed by the administration.[15]

These are just a few examples of how the Bush administration has altered the way scientific and technical information is handled by the federal government. These changes have enormous and widespread effects on the practice of science within the government and in society at large:

> They limit what questions scientists and other government staff are allowed to ask.
>
> They place constraints on what methods can be used to seek answers.
>
> They restrict the selection of who is permitted to ask questions, seek answers, or give advice in government agencies.
>
> They suppress findings solely on the basis that they conflict with administration policies.
>
> They sanction misleading and unjustified claims to bolster results that are "approved of" by the administration.
>
> They routinely place ideologically rigid nonscientist supervisors in charge of government scientific research programs.
>
> They have a chilling effect on the scientific community by exacting retribution, including dismissals, against scientists who ask unapproved questions or produce unapproved-of results.[16]

INCONVENIENT FACTS

In retrospect, there were ominous signs from the start that George W. Bush had little use for "inconvenient" factual information—whether strictly scientific or otherwise. On the campaign trail Bush appeared notably disinterested in policy details and highly selective in the often misleading factual examples he offered. His numbers frequently didn't add up, and he didn't bother to correct them when the discrepancies were brought to his attention. Equally troubling, when the bitterly divisive 2000 election between Bush and Al Gore hit a stalemate in the debacle over the disputed Florida voting results, George W. Bush's surrogates argued forcefully against a recount, even going to the Supreme Court to prevent one from being conducted. What kind of candidate for high elected office, the nation might well have asked, would argue *against* conducting the most accurate vote count possible? Sadly, the incident was a harbinger of things to come: eschewing factual and expert information would soon become a hallmark of the George W. Bush presidency.

Upon his election, Bush quickly made it clear how his administration would handle scientific information. First, he took an unprecedented eight months to name a science advisor. Then, when Bush finally did name John H. Marburger III—a respected physicist from Brookhaven National Laboratory—the president took the unusual step of symbolically demoting his new science advisor by stripping him of an office in the Executive Office Building and the title of "Assistant to the President." Unlike his recent predecessors, Science Adviser Marburger does not normally report to the president himself but rather must go through White House aides.[17]

Slowly but surely over the course of Bush's first term, a series of defectors began to speak out about the president's contempt for factual information and expert judgment. Former secretary of the Treasury Paul O'Neill recounted, for instance, that when Bush's first speech to a joint session of Congress was being prepared, the president was so "distrustful of the agendas of expert staffers in the various departments" that he removed them from the speechwriting loop. As a result, O'Neill said, Treasury economists had no opportunity to correct Bush's egregious $700 billion understatement of the amount of redeemable U.S. debt—an understatement that conveniently made the president's proposed tax cut more palatable.[18]

In May 2003, when Christine Todd Whitman resigned as head of the Environmental Protection Agency, she lamented to a reporter: "In meetings, I'd ask if there were any facts to support our case. And for that, I was accused of disloyalty!" During the 2004 presidential election Whitman denied having made the statement, but by then other Bush advisers had come forward with similar tales.[19]

Dr. Rosina Bierbaum, for instance, a Clinton administration appointee to the Office of Science and Technology Policy (OSTP) who continued to serve into 2001, recalled that from the start of the Bush administration, "The scientists [who] knew the most about climate change at OSTP were not allowed to participate in deliberations on the issue within the White House inner circle."[20]

Perhaps most persuasive—and disturbing—of all was the 2004 testimony of Richard Clarke, the Bush administration's senior counterterrorism adviser on the National Security Council until 2003 and a national security adviser to three previous presidents as well. In 2004, he wrote that, immediately following the terrorist attacks in the United States on September 11, 2001, President Bush became fixated on retaliating against Iraq even though there was no factual evidence that the regime of Saddam Hussein had anything to do with the plane attacks. As Clarke recalls: "The president dragged me into a room with a couple of other people, shut the door, and said, 'I want you to find whether Iraq did this.' Now, he never said, 'Make it up.' But the entire conversation left me in absolutely no doubt that George W. Bush wanted me to come back with a report that said Iraq did this."[21]

Clarke reviewed all available intelligence data and found virtually no link between Iraq and the Al Qaeda terrorist network. But, even on such a vital security matter, the facts didn't impinge on the Bush administration's preset determination. As Clarke explains: "We got together all the FBI experts, all the CIA experts. We wrote the report. We sent the report out to CIA and found FBI and said 'Will you sign this report?' They all cleared the report. And we sent it up to the president and it got bounced by the National Security Advisor or Deputy. It got bounced and sent back saying, 'Wrong answer. . . . Do it again.'"[22]

A TOXIC MIXTURE FOR SCIENCE POLICY

One has to wonder why George W. Bush takes such an antagonistic stance toward the nonpartisan business of gathering and analyzing scientific and technical information. Despite all that has been written about the lack of scientific integrity in the Bush administration, the president's motivation remains open to speculation. After all, scientific and technical information informs political decisions, but never mandates them. The Bush administration could presumably justify its opposition to caps on greenhouse gas emissions on economic grounds, for instance, without resorting to the distortion and censorship of the government's scientific reports on climate change.

By way of explanation, some critics contend that Bush's long years as a lackluster underachiever at some of the nation's most prestigious schools bred in him the pronounced brand of swaggering anti-intellectualism he displays today. According to this theory, Bush's experiences in college, business school, and the private sector led him to such vehement disdain for the liberal elitist establishment that it would virtually define his governing style.[23]

Others, such as Ron Suskind, who has written extensively about the Bush administration, emphasize Bush's born-again Christian religious beliefs. Calling this a "faith-based presidency," Suskind suggests that Bush's religious beliefs place little value on open debate and dialogue. Suskind quotes Bruce Bartlett, a Republican policy adviser to Ronald Reagan and a former Treasury official, who noted that George W. Bush "dispenses with people who confront him with inconvenient facts," because, as Bartlett puts it, "he truly believes he's on a mission from God. Absolute faith like that overwhelms a need for analysis."[24]

While these psychological and religious factors arguably play a role in the Bush administration's approach to policymaking, there is also little doubt that many administration policies reflect straightforward influence peddling and cronyism. Bush has strong and deep ties both to the religious right and to many powerful leaders in the energy industry, and he has afforded both constituencies unprecedented access to the policy-making process in his administration.

The view that the administration's ties to industry explain many of its policy stances is given added credence by the almost Orwellian cynicism in the language Bush policymakers often choose for their proposals: a "Clear Skies Initiative" that undermines the emission regulations of the original Clean Air Act, a "Healthy Forests Act" that increases private logging on public lands.

Particularly troubling in this respect are administration officials' frequent espousals of their commitment to "sound science." As the public health researchers Stanton Glantz and Elisa Ong have chronicled in detail, the call for "sound science," the use of the term itself, has the most cynical of corporate roots, pioneered by the tobacco lobby. Using documents procured in litigation against the tobacco companies, Glantz and Ong show that, in the early 1990s, cigarette companies formed a coalition designed to challenge every aspect of government science, from its studies of global warming to auto safety. They called their group, formed in 1993, "The Advancement of Sound Science Coalition."

As Glantz and Ong explain: "The 'sound science' movement is not an indigenous effort from within the profession to improve the quality of scientific discourse, but reflects sophisticated public relations campaigns controlled by industry executives and lawyers whose aim is to manipulate the standards of scientific proof to serve the corporate interests of their clients."[25] Given its dubious origins, it is telling indeed that "sound science" has been so readily adopted as a rallying cry by top officials in the Bush administration.

Whatever the underlying reasons, there is little question that the Bush administration has created a toxic environment for science policy and technical analysis. As the evidence presented in the ensuing chapters shows, the current politicization of the federal government's handling of scientific and technical information has set the nation on a dangerous path that

> *impoverishes the policymaking process* by leading to choices that are not informed by the best available scientific and technical knowledge;
>
> *weakens our democracy* by denying citizens the benefit of a full and open debate on vital policy matters;
>
> *demoralizes the legions of dedicated career researchers* in the federal government who compile and analyze information; and, ultimately,
>
> *undermines the tradition of scientific and technical excellence* upon which the credibility of our government depends.

Recent surveys offer striking evidence that a significant number of researchers at federal agencies feel their integrity has been compromised. For example, one in five agency scientists at the U.S. Fish and Wildlife Service reported that they have personally been "directed to inappropriately exclude or alter technical information from USFWS scientific documents." The practice has certainly impeded the government's protection of many endangered species. Similarly, a significant majority—some 58 percent—of scientists at the National Oceanic and Atmospheric Administration's Fisheries Department reported that they personally knew of cases where high-level Bush administration appointees in the Commerce Department had "inappropriately altered NOAA Fisheries determinations."[26]

A separate survey, conducted by the Washington, DC–based Public Employees for Environmental Responsibility, asked federal staff at the Environmental Protection Agency's Region 8 office in Denver, Colorado, a series of questions about their agency. Among the findings: some 78 percent of the professional staff surveyed—many of whom are staff scientists—agreed or strongly agreed with the statement that "political interests affect key decisions made by EPA more than they did five years ago."[27]

Results like these lend credence to a rising chorus of concern from many quarters about the conduct of scientific business at federal agencies. Lewis Branscomb, a Harvard University physicist who directed the National Bureau of Standards in the Nixon administration, for example, notes that President Nixon never "hand-picked ideologues to serve on advisory committees, or dismissed from advisory committees very well-qualified people if he didn't like their views. What's going on now," Branscomb says, "is in many ways more insidious. . . . I don't think we've had this kind of cynicism with respect to objective scientific advice since I've been watching government, which is quite a long time."[28]

In response to such charges, White House press secretary Scott McClellan stated in August 2003: "This administration looks at the facts, reviews the science, and then makes a decision, based on that information, that is in the best interest of the American people."[29] All too often, however, as we shall see, a close review of the record reveals a dramatically different story.

2

"Icing" the Data on Climate Change

> In my 14 years in government I have never seen a situation like the present one involving climate science in which politicization by the White House has fed back directly into the science program in such a way as to undermine the credibility and integrity of the program in its relationship to the research community, to program managers, to policymakers, and to the public interest.
>
> RICK S. PILTZ, former senior associate at the U.S. Climate Change Science Program, in his letter of resignation, 2005

The melting of the polar ice caps may be a remote and gradual affair, but nothing is remote or gradual about the Bush administration's attempts to sweep global warming science under the White House rug. The issue of global climate change puts the suppression and distortion of governmental scientific research into stark relief.

Let's look first at the science.

The earth is warming at an unprecedented rate and human activity is largely to blame. That, in a nutshell, is the almost unanimous scientific consensus about global climate change—and it has been since at least 2001, when a landmark review was published by an international panel of leading climate experts.[1] The phenomenon is well understood: the burning of fossil fuels (among other factors) causes what are called greenhouse gases (principally carbon dioxide, plus methane, nitrous oxide, and so-called fluorocarbons) to get trapped in the atmosphere, where they function to warm the planet much as the glass of a greenhouse helps it retain heat in winter. According to scientists' best estimates, mean temperatures for the earth as a whole will rise between 2 and 10 degrees Fahrenheit over the rest of this century.[2] Without concerted human intervention to try to correct or at least stabilize this trend, the world's scientific experts on the subject contend that the pace of global warming will increase dramatically in coming years, with a host of disruptive and possibly devastating consequences to the earth's population, from coastal flooding, caused by a rising sea level, to an increase in powerful hurricanes.[3]

For more than a decade, this consensus about global climate change in the international scientific community has developed as solid, peer-reviewed scientific research has repeatedly and consistently documented changes in the makeup of the atmosphere, the melting of polar ice caps, shifts in the migratory patterns of birds, and a host of other troubling indicators. The popular press, with its penchant for "dissenting" voices, often obscures just how robust this consensus is. Naomi Oreskes, a science historian at the University of California, San Diego, for example, closely reviewed the scientific literature for scientific papers on global climate change published between 1993 and 2003. Of the nearly one thousand scientific articles Oreskes reviewed, *not one* explicitly disagreed with the consensus view that humans are contributing to global warming.[4]

Largely because of the strength of the scientific evidence now on the table, leaders of nearly all of the world's governments, some 141 nations, have signed the so-called Kyoto Protocol—a worldwide effort to curb greenhouse gases.[5] The list of signatories does not, however, include the United States, the world's largest greenhouse gas producer and greatest culprit in global warming. The Bush administration, with its strong ties to the oil and gas industries and its disdain for regulation, staunchly resists the notion that the government should require polluters to curb their carbon emissions. Early in his first term, President Bush reneged on the U.S. commitments to the Kyoto Protocol made by previous administrations. In a statement from the White House in June 2001, Bush called the Kyoto Protocol "fatally flawed." He said the Kyoto mandates to gradually lower emissions of greenhouse gases would have "a negative economic impact" on the United States and that "most reasonable people will understand that it's not sound public policy."[6]

By abandoning the international efforts represented by the Kyoto Protocol—especially as brusquely and abruptly as he did—Bush went against the overwhelming preponderance of international scientific expertise and advice on the subject.

As I have noted, decisions like this exist at the intersection of science and politics. There is no doubt that political considerations will be—and should be—taken into account. But in technical matters such as global climate research, science has a vital role to play: to offer the best, most accurate data possible to help inform the policymaking process.

Considered in this light, Bush administration officials could have furthered their stance in a forthright manner. They could have welcomed any and all new scientific evidence on the issue while explaining to the U.S. public and the world their position that, *despite the scientific evidence,* they believed economic and political considerations dictated continued U.S. inaction on the issue.

This is not the course taken by the Bush administration, and herein lies the most vexing and insidious aspect of the story. Shortly after taking office, President Bush and his staff were confronted with a mounting pile of scientific evidence showing that the earth is, in fact, warming as a result of human-made greenhouse gas emissions. How did the Bush administration respond to this evidence?

MEET PHILIP COONEY

To appreciate the campaign to distort climate change science, let us consider the case of Philip Cooney. From 2001 until 2005, Cooney was chief of staff for the White House Council on Environmental Quality (CEQ). A major part of his job, the evidence shows, was to censor and distort government reports so as to raise doubts about climate change even when U.S. government scientists had none.

Cooney, a lawyer with a bachelor's degree in economics, had no scientific credentials that might qualify him for his position, much less to rewrite the findings of top government scientists. But he did bring a good deal of professional experience that became relevant to the job. Before coming to the Bush administration in 2001, Cooney had spent roughly a decade as a lawyer for the American Petroleum Institute, the oil industry's leading lobbyist in Washington. His last assignment before moving to the council, as so-called climate team leader, was to try to prevent the U.S. government from entering into any kind of international agreement or enacting any domestic legislation that might enforce limits on greenhouse gas emissions.[7] When Cooney joined the White House staff, he pretty much continued to pursue oil industry goals, only with a lot more clout. As chief of staff at the Council on Environmental Quality, however, Cooney represented the U.S. federal government, not the oil industry. His salary was paid by U.S. taxpayers.

During his tenure, Cooney altered numerous official scientific reports on climate change issued by federal agencies, despite his lack of scientific expertise. As U.S. government scientists in the Climate Change Science Program (CCSP), the nation's top interagency program on the issue, struggled to finalize their strategic plan in 2002, for example, Cooney dramatically altered the document they had prepared. Among other interventions, he deleted paragraphs discussing how global warming will reduce mountain glaciers and snowpack in some areas, thereby reducing the availability of water. In the October 2002 draft of the Strategic Plan, the U.S. government's climate scientists had written:

> Warming will also cause reductions in mountain glaciers and advance the timing of the melt of mountain snow packs in polar regions. In turn, runoff rates will change and flood potential will be altered in ways that are currently not well understood. There will be significant shifts in the seasonality of runoff that will have serious impacts on native populations that rely on fishing and hunting for their livelihood. These changes will be further complicated by shifts in precipitation regimes and a possible intensification and increased frequency of extreme hydrological events.[8]

Apparently, the Bush administration wanted to keep this scientific assessment from the U.S. public; Cooney excised it in its entirety. When he wasn't deleting the climate scientists' work, Cooney edited it heavily, repeatedly inserting qualifying words to enhance the sense of scientific uncertainty about climate change and its implications. In two rounds of heavy editing, Cooney ordered an estimated *650 changes* to this report alone.[9]

Subsequently, Cooney ordered roughly a hundred changes in the CCSP's 2003 annual report, *Our Changing Planet*. In virtually every instance, these changes altered or deleted text about the government's research activities and added an appearance of uncertainty to explanations of what climate scientists were learning about the relationship between the buildup of greenhouse gases, climate changes, and impacts on the earth's ecosystems. As just one example, CCSP scientists and staff had written: "Many scientific observations indicate that the Earth is undergoing a period of relatively rapid change." Cooney changed this sentence to read: "Many scientific observations *point to the conclusion* that the Earth *may be* undergoing a period of relatively rapid change" (emphasis added).[10]

By repeatedly and systematically deleting, distorting, or diluting their work on climate change, Cooney angered many government scientists. They found it hard to stomach that someone with no scientific credentials and a long-term vested interest in rejecting the science on global warming was perverting their research. As the *New York Times* reporter Andrew Revkin explained, "That Cooney was doing that kind of revision was kind of horrifying to scientists within the government, and that's why they came to me with the documents."[11]

Much of what we know about the extent of Cooney's efforts comes from disclosures made by Rick S. Piltz. In March 2005, after ten years as a policy analyst in the Climate Change Science Program, he resigned in protest over the manipulative practices of the Bush administration. In a lengthy resignation letter, Piltz charged that top officials had worked to "impede forthright communication of the state of climate science and its implications for society."

Piltz documented his charges by releasing not only his letter but also a cache of evidence—email exchanges, draft documents, interagency correspondence—to the nonprofit Government Accountability Project, which in turn made them available to the press. As his evidence made clear, the changes ordered by political overseers in the Bush administration "tended to alter or delete references to potential public health impacts, the importance of focusing research at the regional level, the relevance of social science involvement, the potential for major changes (e.g., in the Arctic), and the value and significance of climate models and their projections." Furthermore, Piltz said, there were indications that the interference was becoming even more extensive in Bush's second term.

Piltz's resignation letter offered a lengthy list of specific instances of censorship and distortion by top Bush officials, but he devoted special attention to the role of Philip Cooney. As Piltz asks pointedly: "Why are administration political officials who are not career science program managers, and whose job is essentially to satisfy the administration's constituencies on climate change politics and policy, participating in governing the Climate Change Science Program? In particular, why does a former oil industry lobbyist have the authority to edit scientific statements developed by career federal science professionals?"[12]

The Bush administration offered no response, but on June 10, 2005, two days after the *New York Times* first reported Piltz's revelations, Cooney resigned. Implausibly, the White House claimed that Cooney's resignation was unrelated to Piltz's disclosures. A deputy spokeswoman for the White House, Dana Perino, announced that Cooney simply wanted to spend more time with his family. "Phil Cooney did a great job and we appreciate his public service and the work that he did, and we wish him well in the private sector," Perino said.[13]

The private sector—specifically the oil industry—seemed happy to have him back; ExxonMobil hired Cooney one week after he left the White House.[14] The news prompted Kert Davies, the U.S. research director for Greenpeace, to quip that "the cynical way to look at [Cooney's return to the oil industry] is that ExxonMobil has removed its sleeper cell from the White House and extracted him back to the mother ship."[15]

A PATTERN OF DISTORTION

Were the case of Philip Cooney an isolated incident, it might be possible to dismiss it as an error or anomaly. But Cooney's work is just one episode in a saga that began shortly after George W. Bush took office. Despite promises by the president that "my administration's climate change policy will be science-based,"[16] as he said after six months in office, the White House has repeatedly and consistently intervened to distort or suppress climate change research findings.

The story begins in January 2001, just days after the inauguration, when a report by the Intergovernmental Panel on Climate Change (IPCC), under the auspices of the United Nations, determined that there was strong scientific evidence of global warming.[17] The 2001 IPCC assessment, drawing upon the research of some of the world's most respected climate scientists, quickly became a standard reference work and solidified scientific consensus about global warming internationally. Unwilling to accept the findings of the IPCC report, however, in May 2001 the Bush White House officially asked the U.S. National Academy of Sciences (NAS) to conduct its own review of the IPCC assessment.[18]

The request for the NAS review was successful as a delaying tactic, but, coming from an administration trying to avoid doing anything about global warming, it was also a high-stakes gamble. The NAS, both independent and nonpartisan, is frequently viewed by government officials as a kind of final arbiter on scientific matters. John Marburger, Bush's science adviser, even referred to the NAS as the "gold standard" of scientific advice to the government, a view shared by many U.S. scientists and policymakers.[19] It would appear that the Bush administration hoped the NAS panel would raise doubts about the international scientific consensus that greenhouse gases were causing global warming. Contrary to these hopes, however, the panel rendered a swift and strong judgment a month later, in June 2001, confirming the conclusions of the IPCC that global warming was occurring and that the change was linked to industrial greenhouse gas emissions.[20]

To its discredit, the Bush administration responded by largely ignoring the NAS findings it had asked for, as it had ignored the IPCC assessment. The administration continued to contend that scientific uncertainties in climate projects and fossil fuel emissions were too great to warrant action on the issue.[21]

If the White House hoped to keep the issue from public attention, it was to no avail. A year later, in May 2002, the Environmental Protection Agency (EPA) and the State Department released the "U.S. Climate Action Report," which had been required by the United Nations as part of the Clinton administration's participation in worldwide negotiations to respond to global warming.[22] In this report, government scientists pointed to a clear human role in the accumulation of heat-trapping gases, and they detailed the likely negative consequences of climate change, such as the prospect of periods of drought in the Great Plains of the United States.

The report gave the U.S. press cause to question the Bush administration's continued inaction on the issue of global warming. Confronted by the powerful conclusions of influential U.S. government scientists, President Bush responded by disparaging the findings. He called it a "report put out by the bureaucracy," thereby denigrating years of work by scientists throughout the federal government.[23]

After that uncomfortable incident, as Jeremy Symons, a former climate policy adviser at EPA has astutely noted, "The administration took a much bolder approach to dodge such embarrassment: it began to try to minimize awareness of the threat of global warming."[24] A powerful example of this tougher strong-arm strategy to stifle scientific information about climate change occurred in April 2003. In this case, the Bush administration tried to force EPA to substantially alter a section on climate change in the agency's draft *Report on the Environment*—the government's most comprehensive annual environmental assessment.

Philip Cooney and his boss, James Connaughton, at the White House Council on Environmental Quality and John Graham at the Office of Management and Budget demanded a host of major amendments, as internal EPA memos leaked to the press reveal. The draft EPA report had referenced the NAS review and other studies showing that human activity contributes significantly to climate change. These top officials ordered EPA to remove any reference to the NAS report—even though the White House had requested it in the first place. Instead, they demanded that the report refer to a discredited study of temperature records that had been funded in part by the American Petroleum Institute.[25]

The White House also told EPA scientists to delete a temperature record covering one thousand years and documenting a worsening warming trend. As an internal EPA memo put it, the purpose of the deletion was to emphasize instead "a recent, limited analysis [which] supports the administration's favored message." White House officials even ordered the elimination of the report's summary statement—noncontroversial within the climate science community—that "climate change has global consequences for human health and the environment."[26]

Such dramatic additions and deletions weren't the only form of administration interference in the EPA report. White House officials demanded so many qualifying words—such as "potentially" and "may"—that the result, according to the assessment offered in internal EPA documents, would have been to insert "uncertainty . . . where there is essentially none."[27]

Christine Todd Whitman, the EPA administrator at the time, has since described the political climate as "brutal."[28] Ultimately, Whitman, in consultation with the top scientists at EPA, opted to delete the entire section on climate change from the EPA's annual assessment.[29] According to internal EPA documents and interviews with EPA researchers, the agency staff chose this path rather than compromise its credibility by misrepresenting the scientific consensus. Doing otherwise, as one high-ranking EPA official put it, would have "poorly represent[ed] the science and ultimately undermine[d] the credibility of the EPA and the White House."[30]

The EPA's decision to delete any mention of global warming from its report drew immediate attention and criticism because earlier versions of the report—including the climate change section—had already circulated to some members of the press. Many scientists and public officials—Republicans and Democrats alike—decried the administration's political manipulation of scientific inquiry.

The following month, May 2003, Whitman resigned as the head of the U.S. Environmental Protection Agency. At the time, Whitman denied she was leaving because of clashes with the White House, but emails and White House documents that surfaced as part of a Freedom of Information Act request by the attorneys general of Connecticut, Maine, and Massachusetts tell a different story. Trouble was brewing, it seems, for nearly a year. In June 2002, after the administration's embarrassment over the "U.S. Climate Action Report," White House officials sought help to discredit the EPA from Myron Ebell, a conservative lobbyist whose Competitive Enterprise Institute has received over $1 million from ExxonMobil since 1998.[31] The Competitive Enterprise Institute bills itself as an independent think tank, and Ebell and his colleagues pose as full-time, independent technical experts on the issue, writing nay-saying editorials and appearing on panels denying evidence of global warming. Ebell is an economist, not a scientist, but even more than his lack of a scientific background in the climate change field, the fact that Ebell's work is almost entirely underwritten by ExxonMobil—one of the world's largest single greenhouse gas emitters and perhaps the most vociferous corporate voice against governmental climate change regulation—seriously undercuts his credibility. Nonetheless, Ebell worked closely with Philip Cooney, chief of staff at the White House Council on Environmental Quality.

In an email exchange, Ebell and Cooney discussed possible tactics not only for playing down the "U.S. Climate Action Report" but also for getting rid of EPA officials—including Whitman. As Ebell wrote: "It seems to me that the folks at the EPA are the obvious fall guys and we would only hope that the fall guy (or gal) should be as high up as possible."

Ebell urged that the president distance himself from the report, which, of course, Bush subsequently did. "Perhaps tomorrow," Ebell added, "we will call for Whitman to be fired."[32]

A CHILLING EFFECT ON WARMING

To climate scientists, the abuses of the Bush administration are blatant and brazen. They see an administration that embeds industry lobbyists in key regulatory positions; that has so little care for the integrity of scientific data that it routinely distorts and manipulates the findings of government scientists; and that colludes with industry shills to undermine its own government officials. From the start, despite the widespread scientific consensus that human activity and global climate change are connected, the Bush administration has sought to exaggerate and misuse peripheral points of uncertainty and legitimate debate. It has distorted and suppressed scientific and technical analysis on global climate change so as to avoid fashioning any policies that would significantly reduce the threat implied by those findings.

The Bush administration's record on climate change has potentially disastrous consequences for the long-term health of the environment and the generations to come, but the damage to the integrity of the government's scientific research in this field has been significant and much more immediate in its effects.

Scientists and officials who have followed this issue closely understand what is at stake. Russell Train, for instance, served as EPA administrator under presidents Nixon and Ford. Writing in the *New York Times,* Train complained that the Bush administration's actions undermined the independence of the EPA and were virtually unprecedented for the degree of their political manipulation of the agency's research. The "interest of the American people lies in having full disclosures of the facts," Train wrote. As he put it, "I can state categorically that there never was such White House intrusion into the business of the EPA during my tenure."[33]

As a current EPA official puts it, "This administration seems to want to make environmental policy at the White House. I suppose that is their right. But the American public has to ask: On the basis of what information is this policy being promulgated? What views are being represented? Who is involved in the decision making? What kind of credible expertise is being brought to bear?"[34]

Another government scientist told me that one of the most notable things about the Bush administration is how effective it has been at "knowing where the levers of government are" and using them to keep tight control over federal research and assessment.[35] It is a sentiment I have heard echoed repeatedly in one form or another by sources in the federal government.

To see this tight control in action, one need look no further than the case of James E. Hansen, director of NASA's Goddard Institute for Space Studies and one of the world's foremost climate experts. Hansen has frequently been an outspoken critic of the Bush administration's handling of scientific and technical information on climate science. For instance, in 2004 he noted: "In my more than three decades in government, I have never seen anything approaching the degree to which information flow from scientists to the public has been screened and controlled as it is now."[36]

But things for Hansen came to a head in January 2006 when he risked his job by charging publicly that the Bush administration had attempted to silence him after he gave a lecture calling for reductions in greenhouse gas emissions. According to Hansen, a young public affairs officer at NASA named George Deutsch had turned away members of the press when they requested interviews about Hansen's research.

As the full story emerged, it came to light that the twenty-four-year-old Deutsch was, in effect, serving as the administration's censor for NASA's top climate scientist. Deutsch told his colleagues he was doing so because it was his job to "make the president look good." Not only did Deutsch lack credentials in the field to pass judgment on the work of a scientist of Hansen's stature, he quickly resigned in disgrace shortly after this incident was publicized when it was discovered that he had never even graduated from college despite listing a degree from Texas A&M University on his resume.[37]

In the aftermath of this embarrassment to the Bush administration, NASA director Michael D. Griffin issued a statement explicitly calling for openness. "It is not the job of public-affairs officers," Dr. Griffin wrote, "to alter, filter or adjust engineering or scientific material produced by NASA's technical staff."[38] And yet, in the ensuing months scientists at NASA and other agencies, including the National Oceanic and Atmospheric Administration (NOAA), have lodged complaints similar to Hansen's. Much of the problem, they say, stems from the Bush administration policy requiring that all media requests be cleared through central public affairs offices. Officials in these offices, these experts say, routinely stymie and delay such requests, thereby filtering the information the public receives. The result, as Thomas Delworth, a researcher at NOAA's Geophysical Fluid Dynamics Laboratory explained, is that, in the area of climate science, Americans have only "a partial sense" of what the nation's scientists have learned about the subject. "American taxpayers are paying the bill," Delworth asserts; "they have a right to know what we're doing."[39]

To successfully execute tight control over scientific information throughout the federal government is no small feat, yet the Bush White House deems no area too inconsequential for review. Consider, for instance, an incident involving the U.S. Department of Agriculture's Natural Resources Conservation Service (NRCS). In September 2003, this little-known governmental agency sought to reprint a popular informational brochure about "carbon sequestration" in the soil or, in other words, how farmers can help reduce greenhouse gas emissions by reducing their use of energy-intensive fertilizers and pesticides. According to a current government official familiar with the incident, many scientists considered the agency brochure to be a successful effort to discuss climate change. By 2004, the NRCS had distributed some 325,000 brochures, and it was seeking a modest update, as well as proposing a Spanish edition.[40]

This routine proposal went to the White House Council on Environmental Quality for review. William Hohenstein, a Bush official in the office of the chief economist at the USDA, acknowledged that he passed the request on to the CEQ, as he says he would "for any documents relating to climate change policy." Hohenstein denies that he was ever explicitly ordered to do so; rather, he says, he simply knows that the White House is concerned "that things regarding climate change be put out by the government in a neutral way." Presumably because the brochure tacitly accepted the science of global warming, the CEQ objected. As Hohenstein explains, the NRCS ultimately dropped its proposal for a reprint.[41]

"It is not just a case of micromanagement, but really of censorship of government information," a current government official notes. "In nearly fifteen years of government service, I can't remember ever needing clearance from the White House for such a thing."[42]

What is perhaps most notable in the Bush administration's handling of climate change data is the extent to which top Bush officials clearly viewed the emerging scientific research, some of which was gathered by the government's own scientists, as extremely bad news that would be likely to put the administration on the defensive. So, from the start, these officials tried to "put a lid" on this evidence—that is to say, to shut down as much of the government's public disclosure of its scientific research as possible. What research Bush administration officials could not suppress, nonscientists tried to distort and thereby defuse. And when even that strategy didn't work, the administration and its allies and surrogates resorted to demeaning not just the evidence but the scientists who produced it.

In retrospect, we can only infer that, for top officials of the Bush administration, the goal of promoting the economic interests of energy and related industries trumped scientific evidence *no matter what it might suggest.* It is not farfetched to imagine that such a view represented explicit political payback to well-heeled Bush supporters from the energy industry. But it is also true that the many administration officials who have worked or lobbied for—or owned sizable stakes in—energy companies were perhaps in a certain sense "paying themselves back." After all, both President Bush and Vice President Dick Cheney were the heads of oil companies and apparently were importing their highly partisan and cynical industry perspective about climate science into the White House. Top officials throughout the Bush administration formerly worked at, lobbied for, or legally represented the energy industry. Secretary of State Condoleezza Rice, a former director of Chevron, even had an oil tanker named after her—before Chevron quietly rechristened it after she joined the Bush cabinet.

Whatever the origin of the Bush administration's views on the matter, the pertinent point is that these top officials apparently wouldn't want the U.S. federal government to intervene even if millions of the earth's inhabitants were indisputably headed toward imminent and avoidable disruption, dislocation, and destruction. For the Bush administration, it seems, government regulation to ameliorate global warming is simply antithetical to its core values—and to the vested interests of some of its most important constituents and contributors.

It is one thing to be fixed in one's political position. It is quite another to twist and stifle the scientific facts about a situation to serve political ends, but this is what Bush administration officials have done. They tried to hide the truth: that virtually all of the world's reputable climate scientists are convinced that human-caused emissions of carbon dioxide and other heat-trapping gases are making a discernible—and potentially devastating—contribution to global warming. In so doing, the White House engaged in an active campaign of disinformation to mislead the American public.

One of the most worrisome outcomes is the chilling effect that is created by this intrusion of politics into the business of scientific analysis and assessment. This occurred in Rick Piltz's department, the Climate Change Science Program. His office, Piltz says, "quickly adapted to engaging in a kind of anticipatory self-censorship on this and various other matters seen as politically sensitive under this administration." According to Piltz, this self-censorship on the part of career professionals was one of the most "deleterious influences of the administration on the CCSP."[43]

Tim Barnett, a climatologist at the California-based Scripps Institution of Oceanography, agrees. "I've worked in and around Washington for thirty-five years and have never seen middle-level science people so afraid to diverge from administration positions," he says. He adds that Bush's distortions on climate change "are not only irresponsible but a clear and present danger."[44]

In sum, while the Bush administration's political position on climate change may be cause for legitimate debate, its strategy of disinformation and intimidation is deeply and undeniably deceitful. It undermines the U.S. scientific and technical enterprise, which is based upon trust that practitioners will honestly collect data and dispassionately analyze and disseminate it *no matter what the implications*. Equally importantly, the Bush administration strategy strikes at the very heart of our democracy because good decisions can only be made by a well-informed public.

Censorship and the falsification of data are tactics of criminals and despots. They are the methods employed, for instance, by the tobacco industry, whose officials colluded for years to hide the truth they were learning about the deadly public health threat posed by its products. Suppressing and distorting scientific research should never be allowed to become the policy of the U.S. federal government. And this is why the Bush administration's efforts to suppress and manipulate scientific research on climate change ought to be exposed and vociferously denounced no matter what political views one holds. As Chris Mooney, a prolific chronicler and critic of science policy at the Bush White House has said, "There should be a special circle in hell for people who mess with scientific data."[45]

In the end, Piltz's resignation letter puts it best:

> The ability of our society and our elected officials to make good decisions about climate change and numerous other important public issues depends on a free, accurate, honest, and unimpeded flow of communications about the findings of scientific research and scientifically based assessments of relevant issues. To block, distort, or manipulate this flow of communications in order to further political agendas can be seen as analogous to interference with freedom of the press. The White House should not be in the business of pre-clearing scientific communications based on political impact, any more than it should be in the business of pre-clearing the reporting of the news.

The nation benefits from Rick Piltz's courage in speaking out, but he had to leave the government to tell the truth. This is a shame because, as the planet and the issue of climate change continue to heat up, Piltz is precisely the kind of fair broker of scientific information that the government needs.

3

Doctoring Evidence about Your Health

> I expect the Bush administration will go down in history as the greatest disaster for public health and the environment in the history of the United States.
>
> SENATOR JAMES M. JEFFORDS (Independent-VT), 2004

The old adage says, "If it ain't broke, don't fix it." But what if it *is* "broke" and you still don't want to fix it? For the Bush administration, the answer appears to be "doctor" the facts. Such was the case in December 2003 with the release of the *National Healthcare Disparities Report,* the first annual review of its kind, mandated by Congress in 1999 as part of a national effort to eliminate health-care disparities between different racial and ethnic groups.[1] The episode, now largely forgotten, reveals much about the Bush administration's politically motivated manipulation of scientific information.

Sadly, disparities in the availability and quality of health care between different racial and ethnic groups—as well as between the rich and the poor—plague the U.S. health-care system. In one of the more disgraceful examples, black infants are twice as likely to die before the age of one as are white children, a disparity that has lasted for decades.[2] As government scientists and policy analysts investigated the question of disparities, they uncovered a host of troubling facts: racial and ethnic minorities are more likely than whites to be diagnosed with late-stage cancer; they are more likely to die of HIV/AIDS; they are more often subjected to physical restraints in nursing homes; and—especially prevalent in Hispanic communities—they are more likely to receive suboptimal cardiac care for heart attacks.[3]

If the Bush administration had had its way, though, you would never have learned about any of this from the government. Political appointees at the U.S. Department of Health and Human Services (HHS) deleted all of these facts from the scientific report released by its Agency for Healthcare Research and Quality (AHRQ). The report's final draft retained only milder examples of disparities. You wouldn't have learned, for example, the truth of the government's assessment of the gross disparities in the quality of health care in the United States. Instead, the report featured comparatively innocuous information, such as the fact that "Hispanics and American Indians or Alaska Natives are less likely to have their cholesterol checked."[4]

Why would the Bush administration whitewash a congressionally mandated scientific report? Even more to the point, why would the administration want to doctor the facts about U.S. health care, especially on such a touchy national subject as racial disparities?

Once again, the administration perceived scientific findings as unacceptably "bad news" that might, with the attention of the press and the public, ultimately lead to action on issues it preferred to ignore. But the truly baffling aspect of this story is that the administration would have such a cynical view of the issue that it would authorize the distortion of a scientific report that could otherwise contribute to better health care for millions of Americans.

Whatever the motivation or rationale, the administration's efforts backfired badly. After seeing the politically motivated changes that Bush appointees to the Agency for Healthcare Research and Quality were making to the report, an outraged AHRQ scientist leaked the uncensored version to the press. And once the dramatic discrepancies between the earlier draft and the "authorized" report came to light, Rep. Henry Waxman (D-CA), as chair of the House Committee on Government Reform, ordered an investigation.[5]

Congressional staff found that high-ranking political appointees of the Bush administration within HHS, including members of the Office of the Assistant Secretary for Planning and Evaluation, had knowingly manipulated the work of AHRQ scientists. The information they censored and distorted had been compiled in consultation with experts from the National Institutes of Health, the Centers for Disease Control and Prevention, and other health agencies.[6] According to the investigation, the changes, including those mentioned above, substantially altered the conclusions of government scientists regarding racial disparities in the availability and quality of health care in the United States.

The administration even altered the government scientists' main conclusions. The earlier draft had largely reinforced the findings of an influential study by the Institute of Medicine at the National Academy of Sciences that had found "overwhelming" evidence of racial disparities.[7] The December 2003 AHRQ report "minimized the importance and scope of disparities in healthcare," according to the Congressional investigation. For instance, the AHRQ scientists had written as their first finding: "Inequality in quality persists." Nothing unclear about that. But that direct assessment was replaced with the following: "Americans have an exceptional quality of health care; but some socioeconomic, racial, ethnic, and geographic differences exist." The scientists' second finding initially read: "Disparities come at a personal and societal price." This finding was altered to read: "Some 'priority populations' do as well or better than the general population in some aspects of health care." And so on.[8]

Not surprisingly, in a presidential election year, the revelations about the *National Healthcare Disparities Report* made for good partisan fodder. Terry McAuliffe, the chair of the Democratic National Committee, jumped at the chance to state the obvious: "It seems like President Bush and [Health and Human Services] Secretary Tommy G. Thompson have found an easy way to take care of the health disparities faced by minorities," McAuliffe quipped. "They just don't report them."[9]

Following a modest public outcry over the matter and strong protest by members of Congress and some leaders in the scientific community, Thompson did something exceedingly rare for a Bush appointee. He admitted a "mistake." Thompson said in February 2004 that his department was wrong to have revised scientific conclusions in the report, stating that "there was a mistake made, and it's going to be rectified."[10]

Dr. Carolyn Clancy, the director of the Agency for Healthcare Research and Quality, restored the scientists' initial draft to the agency's website. Clancy's explanatory note about the incident, however, was telling. The controversial changes to the draft were made, she wrote, as part of a "routine review."[11] When asked about Clancy's characterization of the changes as "routine," Karen Migdail, a spokesperson for the agency, shed further light on the story. As she put it, because the controversial changes were made as part of "a normal clearance process," the initially released report would most likely have remained unchanged had its earlier version not surfaced.[12] In other words, according to the spokesperson for the agency in question, if a disgruntled federal employee had not leaked the original, uncensored version, the truth—of both the findings of the study and their censoring—would never have come to light.

This is not a comforting thought, given the untold thousands of scientific and technical reports issued under the Bush administration's watch.

LEAD POISONING: MILLIONS OF CHILDREN LEFT BEHIND

The saga surrounding the *National Healthcare Disparities Report* involved a blatant example of distorting the facts. Just as troubling is the Bush administration's calculated strategy to distort the collection of scientific and health information within the government. This begins with the manipulation of the scientific advisory process inside the federal government's network of nearly one thousand scientific advisory panels where new policies often originate and are evaluated on their technical and scientific merits.

Consider what happened in 2002 at the federal Centers for Disease Control and Prevention (CDC) regarding government standards to prevent childhood lead poisoning.

First, a word about the issue at stake. Lead poisoning has long been recognized as a serious threat to children; it can cause brain damage, central nervous system disorders, and many other serious ailments. It is also a classic example of the kind of issue where Americans count on the federal government for guidance and regulation. Since the 1960s, thanks to a variety of federal policies like removing lead from gasoline and most paint, the threat to children from lead poisoning has been reduced substantially. Nonetheless, lead poisoning remains a serious national problem. The CDC estimates that more than four hundred thousand children in the United States under the age of five currently have elevated levels of lead in their blood.[13]

Since the 1970s, as authorized by Congress, the CDC has impaneled a group of experts to advise the government on how to best protect children from lead poisoning. (This is one of roughly two dozen advisory committees within the CDC alone.)[14] The task before the CDC Advisory Committee on Childhood Lead Poisoning Prevention is one of significant consequence: millions of the nation's children, and their parents, depend upon lead poisoning prevention policies based on the best available scientific evidence and technical information. It is also, at least in some measure, thanks to this committee's recommendations that the incidence of elevated lead levels in children has declined significantly over the past several decades.[15]

In the summer of 2002, the Advisory Committee on Childhood Lead Poisoning Prevention was preparing to consider a revision in the federal standard for lead poisoning, which had most recently been set in 1991. Initially, in 1975, the CDC had officially defined "lead poisoning" as the presence of more than 30 micrograms of lead per deciliter of blood. As emerging scientific evidence showed a measurable health threat from exposure to even smaller amounts of lead, the CDC revised its standard. The lead poisoning threshold was lowered in 1985 to 25 micrograms per deciliter and, in 1991, was further reduced to 10 micrograms, where it stands today.[16]

According to numerous sources familiar with the committee's work in 2002, the advisory group was likely to rule in favor of a yet more stringent federal standard for lead poisoning, reflecting the latest research that linked ever-smaller amounts of lead exposure to developmental problems in children.[17] But a few weeks before the committee's meeting to discuss the question, administration officials intervened. Tommy Thompson, then secretary of Health and Human Services, took the unusual step of rejecting nominees selected by the staff scientists of a federal agency under his own jurisdiction. According to Dr. Susan Cummins, who chaired the CDC's lead advisory committee from 1995 to 2000, this was the first time an HHS secretary had ever rejected nominations by the committee or CDC staff.[18] In fact, Thompson's office not only bypassed the respected researchers the CDC staff had recommended, but appointed five new members, forcing the resignation of at least one existing committee member. Even more, all five of the new appointees were on record as opposing a stricter federal lead poisoning standard.[19]

A congressional review soon uncovered what Thompson's office had not mentioned: at least two of the new appointees had financial ties to the lead-paint industry—and thus a direct conflict of interest.[20] One of them, Dr. William Banner Jr., an Oklahoma-based physician, was at the time of his nomination retained by the Lead Industries Association as an expert witness in an ongoing legal case between the state of Rhode Island and lead-paint manufacturers. In that capacity, Banner declared that studies had never adequately demonstrated a link between lead exposure and cognitive problems in children at any level below 70 micrograms per deciliter.[21]

Dr. Banner, a medical toxicologist, also served as an attending physician at Children's Hospital at the University of Oklahoma College of Medicine. But he has not published in the scientific literature on the issue of childhood lead poisoning[22] and holds what most medical specialists on lead poisoning consider a "fringe" view, far from even the normal range of expert scientific discourse. As one medical researcher explains it, Banner's position either ignores or willfully misreads some four decades' worth of accumulating data on the detrimental effects of lead exposure in children.[23]

Researchers may well debate whether the government should tighten its standard for lead poisoning. The public needs and deserves such an informed debate. In this case, however, the Bush administration effectively tampered with the integrity of the advisory panel nominating process, thereby preventing an informed review of the evidence.

To make room for Dr. Banner and the other new appointees, for instance, Secretary Thompson's office dismissed Dr. Michael Weitzman, who had served on the panel for four years. Weitzman, a leading expert on lead exposure, is chief of pediatrics at the University of Rochester School of Medicine and executive director of the American Academy of Pediatrics Center for Child Health Research. Unlike Banner, Weitzman has conducted research on lead exposure and published widely on the subject in peer-reviewed journals. Weitzman states that shortly before he learned of his rejection by Secretary Thompson, CDC staff told him they planned to nominate him to chair the advisory committee.[24]

During the weeks following the controversy over appointments to the committee, an astounding fact came to light: both Banner and another Bush appointee, Dr. Sergio Piomelli, admitted publicly that they were first contacted about serving on the committee by representatives from the lead-paint industry, not by a member of the administration. The industry appeared to be recruiting favorable committee members with the blessing of HHS officials.[25]

The dismissal of Weitzman, the rejection of other CDC-recommended candidates, and the recruitment of industry-selected candidates came via direct intervention from HHS secretary Thompson's office. The blatant intrusion of industry marked a particularly egregious conflict of interest for a scientific panel tasked with helping the federal government protect children's health.

This time, though, unlike the case of the *National Healthcare Disparities Report,* there was no public apology. When asked about his agency's rationale for rejecting scientists selected by their peers and appointing scientific advisers to the government based on the recommendations of industry lobbyists, HHS spokesperson William Pierce stated defiantly that the agency was free to nominate whomever it wanted. Secretary Thompson's staff, Pierce said, "takes into consideration recommendations from people inside and outside of the federal government." Furthermore, Pierce explained, some 258 advisory panels fall under the purview of HHS. At the direction of President Bush, Secretary Thompson planned to "closely and actively oversee" the appointments of scientists to all of them.[26]

No matter what one's political viewpoint, the manner of the administration's intervention into the makeup of the CDC Advisory Committee on Childhood Lead Poisoning Prevention should stand as a troubling tale. The process callously shortchanged all Americans who rely on the federal government to protect the nation's millions of children using the best scientific data available. It offers a textbook example of the vulnerability of the scientific advisory process to overt and excessive political interference. And it illustrates why respect for scientific integrity must lie at the heart of federal policymaking in a democratic society.

"We've seen a consistent pattern of putting people in who will ensure that the administration hears what it wants to hear," says Dr. David Michaels, a research professor in the Department of Environmental and Occupational Health at George Washington University's School of Public Health "That doesn't help science, and it doesn't help the country," adds Michaels, who previously served as assistant secretary for environment, safety, and health at the U.S. Department of Energy during the Clinton administration.[27]

As Michaels points out, it is reasonable to hire political appointees to further a given political agenda, but scientific advisory committees have a distinctly different role: namely, to "advise agencies and the public about what is the best science." When that process becomes politicized, he notes, "the committee's role will be hampered, the nation's best scientists will shun involvement, the government's credibility will suffer, and the public will lose vital input to the government on behalf of its safety and health."[28]

WHEN PUBLIC HEALTH IS A "SENSITIVE ISSUE"

The Bush administration's strategy to politicize the scientific advisory process is so pervasive and problematic that I will review it more fully in chapter 8. There are however, more overt ways to exercise control over the government's agenda on science and health issues. Take, for example, the case of Dr. James Zahn, a research microbiologist at the U.S. Department of Agriculture (USDA). Shortly after joining USDA in 2000, before the start of the Bush administration, Zahn discovered significant levels of antibiotic-resistant bacteria in the air near large hog farms in Iowa and Missouri.[29] He was concerned because the finding suggested that the bacteria could pose a danger to human health, a threat that had not been widely reported elsewhere. Encouraged by his supervisors, Zahn began to study the issue further.

But, Zahn says, the new administration quickly suppressed his research. By focusing on an adverse environmental consequence of hog farming, his work was perceived to be "politically sensitive." Zahn recounts that his superiors repeatedly barred him from publishing his findings or presenting them at scientific conferences in 2002. On no fewer than eleven occasions, he says, he was prohibited from publicizing his research on the potential hazards to human health posed by airborne bacteria resulting from farm wastes.[30] He says he received a message from a supervisor advising him that "politically sensitive and controversial issues require discretion."[31]

In fact, the USDA's effort to control so-called sensitive topics addressed by its research scientists is part of an explicit administration policy. An agencywide directive issued in February 2002 requires all USDA staff scientists to seek prior approval before publishing any research or speaking publicly on any "sensitive issues." According to the memo, sensitive issues include any "agricultural practices with negative health and environmental consequences, e.g. global climate change; contamination of water by hazardous materials (nutrients, pesticides, and pathogens); animal feeding operations or crop production practices that negatively impact soil, water, or air quality."[32]

There is nothing subtle or ambiguous about that directive. In the Bush administration, USDA scientists need special permission to talk about anything involving agricultural pollution of air, water, or soil that might ruffle the feathers of agribusiness. Zahn says USDA officials told him his work was being discouraged because issues affecting human health were "outside his unit's mission." Yet the website for Zahn's research unit at USDA states explicitly that its mission "is to solve critical problems in the swine production industry that impact production efficiency, environmental quality, *and human health*" (emphasis added).[33]

In fact, Zahn says, industry representatives overtly influenced the suppression of his work. In one instance, Zahn recounts, USDA prevented him from addressing a meeting of the Board of Health in Adair County, Iowa. He later found a fax trail showing that the National Pork Producers Council had complained to his boss at USDA after learning of Zahn's scheduled appearance. It was after that intervention that Zahn was denied permission.

Zahn's superiors scolded him for seeking to publicize findings that raised questions about industry practices. But the fact is that Zahn, who had earned his doctorate from Iowa State University and won several major research awards, including one from the American Society for Microbiology, was simply a dedicated research scientist doing exactly what he was hired to do.

Dr. Alan DiSpirito, a microbiologist at Iowa State University, notes that Zahn, with whom he collaborated on related research, was careful never to make unwarranted claims about health effects. As DiSpirito puts it, Zahn "found evidence of airborne toxic substances and antibiotics, which certainly raised health questions, but as a careful and very competent scientist, he never commented on these in his work except to suggest that someone else ought to look into them."[34]

Zahn, who has since left the USDA to work in the agrichemical industry, offers a harsh critique of the agency. He contends that, in the Bush administration, USDA officials routinely exploited the expansive "sensitive issue" directive to stifle controversial research by forcing it through an extended and politicized approval process. In this way, he says, they create "a choke hold on objective research."[35]

WHERE'S THE BEEF?

The administration suppressed James Zahn's research. But it is important to note that the politicization of scientific information can also involve the concerted effort to make the science fit a desired policy. Consider the situation recounted by a high-ranking source at USDA about the manipulation of science in policymaking after a case of mad cow disease—bovine spongiform encephalopathy (BSE)—was discovered in Canada.

In May 2003, Canadian officials announced the discovery of a case of BSE in a single cow in Alberta. The cow and its herd of 150 were quickly destroyed. As required by existing U.S. regulations, USDA immediately ordered the border closed to live and processed cattle, sheep, and goats from Canada.[36] Scientists began investigating the extent of the problem and assessing the risk to the North American beef supply. Meanwhile, enormous trade pressures began to mount to reopen the U.S. market to Canadian beef.

The importation of Canadian beef is a multibillion-dollar business. According to the USDA, Canada exports some $1.1 billion in live cattle and $1.9 billion in beef to the United States.[37] BSE, however, poses a serious threat to human health. By eating parts of infected animals, humans can contract a fatal variant of Creutzfeldt-Jakob disease, the human form of mad cow disease. More than one hundred people around the world have died from this Creutzfeldt-Jakob variant since an outbreak began Europe in the 1980s. There is no known cure.

Despite the potential risks to the American public, by August, less than three months after the Canadian outbreak of BSE, Secretary of Agriculture Ann M. Veneman announced that the United States would begin to open the border to some Canadian beef products. As Veneman explained, "Our experts have thoroughly reviewed the scientific evidence and determined that the risk to public health is extremely low."[38] In fact, according to a top USDA official, the department's risk assessment of the BSE situation had not even been started at the time of Veneman's announcement.[39]

By law, the USDA must conduct a risk assessment when its policy decisions will have an economic impact of $100 million or more.[40] But during September and October 2003, as Veneman's office moved to open the border to more Canadian beef products, the menu of questions put before USDA's risk assessment branch was repeatedly altered to produce results that would support the decision the department had already made, according to this knowledgeable inside source and corroborated by draft documents and internal agency emails he made public relating to the incident.

The purpose of a risk assessment, of course, is to provide policymakers with analytical data as a basis for making decisions. But in this case the department's analysis was requested after the decision. "There is no question," according to this longtime USDA official, that staff were being asked to "do the risk assessment to support the decision that had already been made."[41]

Veneman's August 2003 announcement that the U.S. would reopen the border to some Canadian beef imports drew criticism from a number of consumer groups. As Michael Hansen of Consumers Union told the press: "The administration seems to be more concerned with trade or trade concerns than public health."[42] In light of this source's revelations about the process within USDA, Hansen's critique now appears more accurate than he probably knew.

The issue of concern here is not the extent to which Veneman's decision posed a significant danger to U.S. consumers. Rather, it is the clear threat her decision posed to the integrity of her department's scientific assessment process. The incident illustrates an all-too-common pattern within the Bush administration: scientific assessments, if they are considered at all, are manipulated to conform to preconceived political positions.

In the words of the outraged USDA staffer who came forth with the truth about the process within his department: "Doing risk assessment after the fact rather than to provide a basis for the decision defeats the whole purpose and is an affront to the integrity of the researchers who undertake the analysis."[43]

"SPIN DOCTORS"

Historically, the federal government, recognizing its vital role as a regulator and protector of public health, has worked hard to establish a climate that protects government scientists from outside influence peddlers. These protections have eroded in the Bush administration. On public health issues, the administration has allowed industry concerns to trump those of public health and independent scientific analysis. It did so when it allowed the lead-paint industry to skew the scientific advisory process and when it allowed pork manufacturers to silence a government scientist's environmental concerns. Notably, these disparate actions cannot be explained away as the result of renegade actors. Rather, all of the incidents involved top agency officials, working at the behest of Bush administration appointees as part of explicit administration policy. Through such actions, the Bush administration has undermined the scientific integrity and credibility of the federal agencies in question.

Such effects can also be seen clearly in two high-profile cases at the U.S. Food and Drug Administration (FDA), in which government scientists raised grave concerns about the safety of popular prescription drugs. Falling on the heels of one another, these cases led to widespread criticism of the FDA's safety mechanisms and allegations that the agency had "too cozy" a relationship with pharmaceutical firms. Such allegations have perennially plagued the FDA, but the particulars of these cases illustrate a pervasive climate in which industry concerns predominate, making it difficult for scientists to conduct independent analyses.

In the first case, which began in June 2003, the FDA selected Dr. Andrew Mosholder, a highly credentialed physician and epidemiologist in the agency's Office of Drug Safety, to review data about commonly prescribed antidepressants from twenty-two clinical trials involving over four thousand children. Half a year later, Mosholder discovered a troubling link between antidepressants and suicidal behaviors in children. In fact, his research showed that certain antidepressants could double the risk of such suicidal behavior in this population group.[44]

What happened next led to widespread public concern and spawned two congressional investigations. In February 2004, when Mosholder sought to present his research to a meeting of FDA scientists, his FDA superiors—political appointees of the Bush administration—notified him at the last minute that he could not do so. Anne Trontell, the deputy director of the FDA's Office of Drug Safety, notified surprised participants at the February 2, 2004, meeting that Dr. Mosholder was being removed from the schedule because his work did not constitute "a finalized document."[45] In fact, as the investigations would show, the determination to suppress Mosholder's findings had nothing to do with how "finalized" the research was.

Ultimately, those findings would be thoroughly corroborated and lead both to warning labels on antidepressants and to dramatic decreases in the extent to which they were prescribed to children. But what is most notable here is how his supervisors first greeted Mosholder's controversial research. Not only did they prevent him from sharing it with his scientific colleagues at FDA but, after word of the incident leaked out, the FDA's Inspector General's office threatened Mosholder with criminal charges if he discussed the matter with anyone. Looking back, it seems the agency was more concerned with determining who had leaked information about Mosholder's work than it was in the vital public health issues this respected scientist had raised.[46]

In the second incident, beginning in August 2004, Dr. David Graham, an associate director in the FDA's Office of Drug Safety and a senior safety official at the FDA for twenty years, told his supervisors of disturbing findings about cardiovascular risks in patients taking the popular painkiller Vioxx. Sold by the pharmaceutical firm Merck, Vioxx was a blockbuster prescription drug with sales grossing over $1 billion annually. But Graham's research indicated that Vioxx use significantly increased the risk of cardiac problems. In fact, he found, high-dose prescriptions of Vioxx could *triple* patients' risk of heart attack.

Just as in Andrew Mosholder's case, the most extraordinary part of the story is the way top FDA officials responded to Graham's disturbing findings. They did not rush—or even begin the process—to remove

Vioxx from the market. Instead, they told Graham to be quiet. They tried to stop him from publishing his research. They even tried to get him to resign.

Fearing for his job as he prepared his manuscript for publication, Graham approached the Government Accountability Project (GAP)—a Washington, DC, nonprofit group that helps government whistleblowers. And again, the administration's response was highly suspect. As GAP's legal director Tom Devine later reported, his office received an anonymous phone call saying that Dr. Graham had bullied other staff and that his study was seriously flawed. Tracing the telephone number, Devine found that the call originated from the offices of top FDA management.

When Graham submitted his work to the prestigious British medical journal *The Lancet,* FDA managers tried to force him to pull the article, saying he hadn't first submitted it for an internal review. Devine says this is untrue. In fact, he says, Dr. Graham had sought clearance weeks earlier.[47] Nonetheless, Dr. Lester Crawford, FDA's acting commissioner, criticized Graham for evading the agency's "long-established peer review and clearance process." Worse yet, top Bush appointees at FDA began a smear campaign against Dr. Graham. Dr. Steven K. Galson, the acting director of the drug-evaluation division, told reporters that Graham's work constituted "junk science." Galson even sent an email to an editor at *The Lancet,* trying unsuccessfully to discredit the "integrity" of Graham's data.

Graham persisted in the face of such resistance. In November, after word of his findings had leaked to the public, he appeared before a Senate Finance Committee hearing on Vioxx, where he reported that the drug's use had contributed to some twenty-eight thousand heart attacks in the five years since its introduction in 1999. At the high end of his statistical projections, he testified, the toll Vioxx had already taken was comparable to the roughly fifty-eight thousand Americans killed in Vietnam.[48]

Ultimately, other scientists conducted research that corroborated Graham's findings. Merck removed Vioxx from the market. Furthermore, around the world, medical professionals decried the behavior of the FDA, one of the world's lead drug regulators, for worrying more about protecting industry than protecting public health.

What joins these two episodes is how difficult it was for Mosholder and Graham to get a fair hearing for their research. Government insiders say the overt interference was greatly exacerbated by Bush administration policies. In one notable initiative, for instance, in January 2002 Tommy Thompson, who oversaw the FDA and other health-related agencies as secretary of HHS, issued a directive mandating all federal agency staff "to speak in one voice." As one high-level official warned at the time of Secretary Thompson's directive: "The worst thing [about this plan] is that the people who will be controlling the information flow are going to be spin doctors instead of medical doctors."[49]

Clearly, the notion of "speaking in one voice" is antithetical to creating a climate where government scientists can conduct independent analyses related to matters of vital concern to the American public. As Graham told the Senate Finance Committee in November 2004: "The FDA, as currently configured, is incapable of protecting America against another Vioxx. We are virtually defenseless."[50]

4

Abstaining from the Truth on Abstinence and AIDS

> For the first time in history, the FDA is not acting as an independent agency but rather as a tool of the White House. It is a very sad day when politicians start making medical decisions.
>
> JAMES TRUSSELL, Princeton University scientist and
> FDA advisory committee member, May 2004

No set of issues better encapsulates the Bush administration's antipathy toward facts than its policymaking on matters of human sexuality. From the transmission of AIDS to the prevention of teen pregnancies, Bush administration policies built on empty rhetoric have dispensed outright misinformation to the public and greatly undermined the credibility of the federal agencies involved in public health. Furthermore, when confronted with its programs' abject failures, Bush administration officials have tried to hide the truth, mislead the public, and demean the government researchers seeking to grapple productively with these difficult social issues.

Worst of all is the needless harm Bush administration policies cause to the nation's public health. To date, these policies have unquestionably increased the numbers of Americans requiring abortions, engaging in high-risk, unprotected sex, and contracting sexually transmitted diseases, including AIDS.

Let's begin by looking in greater depth at the way the Bush administration's Food and Drug Administration (FDA) handled issues related to the emergency contraceptive levonorgestrel, sold under the brand name "Plan B."

Plan B consists of two doses of hormones, in pill form that, if taken within seventy-two hours after unprotected sexual intercourse, can prevent pregnancy. Manufactured by New York–based Barr Pharmaceuticals, Inc., Plan B was approved by the FDA as a prescription drug in 1999. Following the agency's thorough evaluation of Plan B's safety and efficacy, millions of women in the United States have safely used it to prevent pregnancy. Virtually all public health officials and researchers around the world agree that Plan B is safe and effective. The drug is available without a prescription in France, the United Kingdom, and more than thirty other countries. Its shift to nonprescription status in the United States has been endorsed by no fewer than seventy scientific organizations, including the American Medical Association, the American College of Obstetricians and Gynecologists, and the American Academy of Pediatrics.[1]

The benefit of emergency contraception such as Plan B, of course, is that it affords a woman the opportunity to avoid an unwanted or unintended pregnancy. In so doing, it also reduces the demand for abortion. Indeed, almost everyone in the polarized debate over abortion politics in the United States—from religious anti-abortion activists to women's rights proponents to the Bush administration—agrees that reducing the demand for abortions is a worthy goal. Even making "morning after" drugs such as Plan B available only on a prescription basis has accounted for some 43 percent of the modest decline in the number of abortions in the United States between 1995 and 2000, according to the Alan Guttmacher Institute, which studies sexual behavior.[2]

As outlined in chapter 1, in December 2003, the FDA voted on Barr Pharmaceuticals' proposal to make Plan B available at pharmacies without out a prescription. The company gained the overwhelming support of a joint meeting of two independent FDA scientific advisory committees, and the vote was 23 to 4 to recommend the emergency contraceptive as an over-the-counter drug. The panels also voted—unanimously—that the drug was safe enough to be sold over the counter.[3]

In an almost unprecedented repudiation of government scientific expertise, however, Steven Galson, then acting director of the FDA's Center for Drug Evaluation and Research, overturned the recommendations of the two FDA advisory panels and of his own staff. He declared the drug "not approvable" for nonprescription status,[4] even though the FDA is required to approve drugs that are found to be safe and effective. Former FDA officials told the *New York Times* they could not remember a single instance when someone in Dr. Galson's position had overruled both advisory committee and staff recommendations. Dr. Robert R. Fenichel, who had left the agency in 2000 after twelve years, for instance, called the action "simply unheard of."[5]

Paul Blumenthal, a respected obstetrician-gynecologist at Johns Hopkins Hospital in Baltimore, noted that Plan B had met all the scientific criteria for an over-the counter drug: it is not toxic, there is no potential for addiction or abuse, and there is no need for medical screening. "What the FDA has just done is deny access to an important pregnancy preventive agent to millions of women," Dr. Blumenthal said about the "not approvable" decision. "This is nothing but politics trumping science."[6]

Why would the Bush administration deny American women easy access to a safe, effective means of emergency contraception that could reduce the demand for abortions? In his "not approvable" letter to Barr Pharmaceuticals, Dr. Galson complained that only 29 of the 585 women in the clinical trial data submitted by the company about Plan B were fourteen to sixteen years of age and none was under fourteen. While Galson did not cite any particular safety concern for this age group, he wrote that "we have concluded that you have not provided adequate data to support a conclusion that Plan B can be used safely by young adolescent women for emergency contraception without the professional supervision of a practitioner licensed by law to administer the drug."[7]

James Trussell calls Galson's argument nothing more than a "scientific fig leaf." Trussell, who is the director of the office of population research at Princeton University and a member of one of the FDA advisory committees that recommended the drug's approval for over-the-counter sale, explains that after hearing many hours of testimony and reviewing thousands of pages of medical literature, "Our committee had absolutely no concern about the use of this drug by young girls."[8] Advisory committee member Dr. Julie Johnson, a professor of pharmacy in Gainesville, Florida, went so far as to state that Plan B was "the safest product the committee had reviewed in several years."[9]

Furthermore, as many medical professionals noted, Galson's objection did not even hold up to scrutiny when taken at face value. The American Academy of Pediatrics and the Society of Adolescent Medicine noted, for instance, that the ratio of participants in the Barr trials between the ages of fourteen and sixteen was consistent with the ratio at which that age group engaged in sexual intercourse relative to the broader population.[10]

FDA advisory panel member Alastair Wood co-wrote an article in the *New England Journal of Medicine* with two colleagues in which he explained that FDA advisory panels had given careful consideration to the issue of label comprehension by adolescent girls. The data the panels reviewed showed that adolescents understood between 60 and 97 percent of the key communication objectives of the Plan B label without help from a health-care professional. The results were comparable to those for all age groups and well within the standards for the approval of over-the-counter drugs.[11]

Dr. Trussell didn't mince words. Galson's action, he said, was "nothing more than a made-up reason intended to sound plausible. From a scientific standpoint, it is complete and utter nonsense."[12] If the advisory committees and the FDA staff didn't share Galson's concerns, where did his objection stem from?

MEET DAVID HAGER

If there is a poster child for the Bush administration's policies on matters of sex and women's reproductive issues, it is Dr. W. David Hager, a Kentucky-based obstetrician and gynecologist who mixes a heavy dose of religious preaching into his medical practice. Hager's nomination to the FDA's Reproductive Health Advisory Committee sent a shockwave through political and scientific circles alike.

Dr. Hager is the author of several books, including *As Jesus Cared for Women: Restoring Women Then and Now* (1998), which recommends scripture readings as a treatment for premenstrual syndrome, postpartum depression, and eating disorders. A staunch anti-abortion activist far out of the mainstream of the medical profession, Hager has publicly likened the contraceptive pill to abortion and, in his private practice, has reportedly refused to prescribe contraceptives to unmarried women.[13]

As press accounts have noted in detail, Hager is an aggressive advocate for the Christian Right's political agenda. As a member of the Christian Medical and Dental Society, for instance, he helped submit a petition to the FDA in August 2002 to halt distribution and marketing of the abortion pill RU-486.

Appointing such a religious extremist to a scientific advisory board on women's reproductive issues was a highly controversial move, even for the Bush administration. To help limit opposition, the administration actually announced Hager's appointment to the panel on Christmas Eve in 2002, ensuring that it would receive little immediate notice in the press.

Hager says he personally refuses to prescribe Plan B to his patients on moral grounds. "Your faith is an integral part of your life and everything that you do," he told a reporter, contending that "83 percent of patients in this country say that they prefer that their physicians pray with them."[14] It also bears noting, given Hager's moralizing about issues of women's sexuality, that he has drawn controversy for his own alleged sexual proclivities. In a recent account, his now-divorced wife, also a devout Christian, asserts that Hager not only cheated on her during their marriage but forcibly sodomized her against her will on a regular basis for at least seven years until she divorced him—in the same year he was appointed to the FDA panel.[15]

Since becoming a government adviser, Hager has taken ample advantage of his position. As a member of FDA's advisory panel, it was Hager who first raised the spurious issue of whether the sample size of young girls in Barr Pharmaceuticals' clinical trials was too small. He brought up the issue at the FDA advisory panel meeting. Then, he says, when a request came "from outside the agency" for a minority report, he followed up with a letter about the issue to Galson.[16] In 2005, speaking to a religious congregation, Hager explained his role in the FDA's decision: apparently he was doing the Lord's bidding as well as George W. Bush's. "God has used me to stand in the breach," Hager told the congregation. He said that when he urged Galson to overturn the panel's recommendations, "I argued from a scientific perspective, and God took that information, and he used it through this minority report to influence the decision."[17]

Hager may have bragged that he argued from a "scientific perspective," but there is little doubt about what really motivates him and the Bush administration to try to block Plan B from being sold over the counter. The objections have little to do with science and everything to do with the politics of right-wing Christian fundamentalists.

First of all, Hager and the Bush administration consider Plan B through the lens of anti-abortion politics. Scientifically speaking, the drug normally works as a contraceptive—that is, it prevents ovulation in the woman who takes it so that conception and pregnancy cannot occur. However, there is a chance that ovulation may have occurred at the time the drug is taken. In that case, within the first seventy-two hours after intercourse, Plan B would prevent the egg's implantation in a woman's uterus. In other words, in some cases the drug could take effect after conception has occurred.

The expressed view of David Hager—and the de facto view of the U.S. government under the Bush administration—is that life begins at the moment of conception and thus Plan B can be equated with abortion. Therefore, Hager believes, it is his moral duty to "save the lives" of these hours-old embryos even though, medically and scientifically, the accepted standard for when a pregnancy begins—according to the Code of Federal Regulations, the American College of Obstetricians and Gynecologists, and the National Institutes of Health, among others—is after implantation in a woman's uterus.

The logic of Hager's—and the Bush administration's—fundamentalist ideology makes it a moral imperative to impose their sectarian view on all women in the United States, even if it realistically means that the number of abortions will surely rise as a consequence.

Arguing for compassion based on the facts, a number of FDA advisory committee members underscored the importance of making recommendations based on a risk-benefit analysis, particularly in regard to young people. Dr. Leslie Clapp, a pediatrician from Buffalo, New York, for instance, spoke about her own clinical practice and acknowledged that, while abstinence is the best option for teens, "If you are a sexually active ten or eleven year old, it's certainly a bad situation. . . . I think their families and they would have far preferred this option than pregnancy, and it would have been safer."[18] Dr. Abby Berenson, a specialist in adolescent gynecology from Galveston, Texas, echoed the sentiment. She argued that "barriers to use," such as a prescription requirement for Plan B, "will ultimately result in unintended pregnancies." These, in turn, pose disproportionate health risks to adolescent women, including premature labor, anemia, and high blood pressure.[19]

Such logic is irrelevant to Hager and senior Bush administration officials because it conflicts with their policy agenda of demonizing the "social ill" posed by sex outside marriage. With regard to the Plan B debate, Hager and top administration officials presumably believe that the availability of an emergency contraceptive without a prescription will lead women to be more promiscuous. It doesn't matter that the facts do not substantiate this concern. Prominent medical studies have shown that there is no link between sexual activity and access to Plan B or other emergency contraceptives. For instance, a recent study in the United Kingdom showed that making emergency "morning after" contraceptive pills available over the counter—as Britain did in 2001—has not changed rates of contraceptive use or unprotected sex.[20] Indeed, as David Grimes of Family Health International noted, it is no more accurate to say that emergency contraception will promote risky sexual behavior than it is to say "that a fire extinguisher beneath the kitchen sink makes one a risky cook."[21]

Were concerns about women's promiscuity behind the bogus objections voiced by FDA's Galson? Some of his own staff seemed to think that's what motivated the Bush administration appointee. After all, Galson broke with agency protocol, not only by overruling two advisory panels and his own staff, but by taking the practically unprecedented step of writing the official response to the drug company himself.[22] In an internal FDA memo obtained by the Associated Press, Galson tried to quell complaints from his own staff. As he noted in that memo: "Some staff have expressed the concern that this decision is based on non-medical implications of teen sexual behavior, or judgments about the propriety of this activity."[23] Answering these concerns, Galson asserted that politics did not influence his decision. He also claimed, in a press conference following his decision, that he had not "met personally" with any White House officials during the decision-making process.[24] But few close watchers of the incident could find these carefully scripted denials much more credible than the bogus scientific objection he had raised in the first place.

After Galson's ruling, Barr Pharmaceuticals swiftly reapplied for FDA approval with a revised proposal to sell Plan B on a nonprescription basis but behind the pharmacy counter so that it could be dispensed only to girls sixteen years or older. In August 2005, the sorry tale seemed to reach a conclusion when the FDA decided to "indefinitely postpone" its decision about Plan B, effectively prohibiting the drug from being sold without a prescription. The issue had been heatedly discussed earlier that year in the Senate confirmation of the Bush administration's since-departed FDA head, Lester M. Crawford, who had promised a final FDA decision on the matter. Crawford's wholly unprecedented move, for the agency to indefinitely withhold nonprescription status for a drug verified as safe and effective by the agency's own scientists, resulted in the resignation of one of FDA's top officials, Susan Wood, director of the agency's Office of Women's Health.[25]

Dr. Frank Davidoff, who was a member of the FDA's Nonprescription Drugs Advisory Committee, also quit the agency. In his resignation letter, Davidoff wrote: "I can no longer associate myself with an organization that is capable of making such an important decision so flagrantly on the basis of political influence rather than the scientific and clinical evidence."[26] Even more recently, in November 2005, a review by the Government Accountability Office confirmed that the incident "did not follow FDA's traditional practices." As the GAO report explains, while the accounts provided by FDA officials differed, there was good evidence to indicate that the decision on Plan B had been made at the highest levels *before the agency's scientific review had been completed.*[27]

PLAYING POLITICS WITH PUBLIC HEALTH

The manipulation of scientific evidence around Plan B tells a sorry tale, but the bigger picture is even more troubling. Since his tenure as governor of Texas, George W. Bush has made no secret of his view that, with regard to sex, teenagers should be taught "abstinence only." Many Bush supporters like the sound of the president's strong pronouncements on these issues, viewing the administration's abstinence-only policies as welcome in a society awash in sexually provocative advertising and entertainment.

To be sure, Bush's notion of "abstinence" is an arguably laudable goal, especially for young teens, but the insistence on "abstinence only" raises deeply troubling issues. Most important, it prevents the government from disseminating information that could help Americans avoid sexually transmitted diseases and pregnancy.

Let's look at the facts.

In the United States, some nine hundred thousand teenagers become pregnant every year. Eight out of ten of these teenagers say their pregnancy was unintended, and there is no doubt that most of these young people are physically, emotionally, and economically ill-prepared for parenthood. Few would deny the merit of federal government policies to try to lower the number of unintended pregnancies among U.S. teenagers. Although the rate of teen pregnancy in the United States decreased somewhat over the 1990s, it is still almost twice that of any other industrialized nation and some ten times higher than it is in the Netherlands or Switzerland.[28]

The incidence of sexually transmitted diseases among teens is also a major public health issue. According to the latest estimates, there are fifteen million new cases of sexually transmitted diseases in the United States each year, and approximately one-quarter of them affect teenagers. Among these diseases, of course, is HIV/AIDS. At the end of 2003, some ten million youths and young adults in the United States were living with HIV/AIDS. In fact, fully one-half of the new HIV infections in the United States and worldwide occur in people under the age of twenty-five.[29]

Despite these disturbing figures, the Bush administration has gutted government programs that offer sex education and increased funding for programs that inculcate "abstinence only." Toward this end, the Bush administration spent approximately $170 million on abstinence-only education programs in 2004, more than twice the amount spent in fiscal year 2001.[30]

What do the administration's favored programs teach? Reviewing the federally sponsored abstinence curricula, a 2004 congressional report offered disturbing answers. According to the report, 80 percent of the abstinence-only curricula supported by the federal government contain false, misleading, or distorted information. Many of the curricula downplay the effectiveness of condoms in preventing sexually transmitted diseases and pregnancy, while greatly exaggerating the dangers posed by abortion.

One curriculum goes so far as to say, for example, that "the popular claim that 'condoms help prevent the spread of STDs,' is not supported by the data."[31] This statement is patently untrue. Another, relying on a thoroughly discredited 1993 study, erroneously states that "in hetero-sexual sex, condoms fail to prevent HIV approximately 31 percent of the time."[32]

With regard to abortion, according to the congressional report, one federally sponsored curriculum states, utterly incorrectly, that 5 to 10 percent of women who have legal abortions become sterile and that "premature birth, a major cause of mental retardation, is increased following the abortion of a first pregnancy."[33]

Equally troubling, the congressional report documents that many of the curricula sponsored by the Bush administration blur the distinction between religion and science. They present as a scientific fact the view that life begins at conception and refer, in one case, to the fetus as a "thinking person."[34] One curriculum even misidentifies the number of chromosomes that join to create a new human being.[35]

It is bad enough that the Bush administration is sanctioning gross distortions and wholesale misinformation. From a purely economic standpoint, the inescapable conclusion is that the Bush administration is pouring hundreds of millions of dollars into programs whose efficacy is dubious at best. To date, *no* abstinence-only education program has been shown to have had any sustainable positive effect on teen pregnancy, sexual activity, or sexually transmitted disease. In the most comprehensive analysis of teen pregnancy prevention programs, researchers found that "the few rigorous studies of abstinence-only curricula that have been completed to date do not show any overall effect on sexual behavior or contraceptive use."[36]

Even Michael Young, a professor of health science at the University of Arkansas and a developer of an abstinence curriculum called "Sex Can Wait," acknowledges that many programs lack published evaluations in peer-reviewed journals. As he puts it, "The amount of money being spent on this is pretty ridiculous when you look at the lack of accountability for outcomes."[37]

George W. Bush's pre–White House experience offers further cause for concern. Texas spent more than $10 million on abstinence-only programs during his tenure as governor—with no discernible curbing of either teen pregnancies or the spread of HIV and other sexually transmitted diseases. Throughout Governor Bush's tenure, from 1995 to 2000, the state ranked last in the nation in the decline of teen birth rates among fifteen- to seventeen-year-old females.[38] Overall, Texas's teen pregnancy rate, with abstinence-only programs in place, was exceeded by only four other states.[39]

Even worse, of course, is the troubling likelihood that abstinence-only programs actually increase health risks. In 2002, for instance, Columbia University researchers reported that while programs that encourage participants to pledge to remain virgins until marriage did help some participants to delay sex, some 88 percent of the participants eventually had premarital sex. When they did have sex, virginity pledgers were less likely to use contraception and less likely to seek testing for sexually transmitted diseases, despite comparable infection rates.[40]

"Think of it this way," a staff scientist at the Centers for Disease Control and Prevention suggested to me. "If the issue were transportation and you were trying to reduce highway fatalities, the Bush administration's policy is to issue gold-plated 'Drive Safely' bumper stickers. That's bad enough as it is, but it becomes literally criminal when the same government denies funding for seat belts and air bags."[41]

A recent newspaper editorial offered a similar assessment: "Teaching a child misinformation about condom failures doesn't stop the child from having sex; it stops the child from using a condom during sex."[42]

EYES WIDE SHUT

Ironically, many studies show that comprehensive sex education that both encourages abstinence *and* teaches about the effective use of contraceptives delays the occurrence of teen sex, reduces the frequency of sex, and increases the use of condoms and other contraceptives. The American Medical Association, the American Academy of Pediatrics, the American Public Health Association, and the American College of Obstetricians and Gynecologists all support comprehensive sex education programs that encourage abstinence while also providing adolescents with information on how to protect themselves against sexually transmitted diseases.[43] Five successive U.S. surgeons general—dating from the early days of the AIDS epidemic—have also endorsed such a comprehensive approach to sex education.[44]

In short, we know a lot about how to prevent pregnancy and sexually transmitted diseases in young people. And one would think that the Bush administration, given the penchant for accountability it promotes through standardized testing in education, for example, or almost any program to help lower-income Americans, would want to test the efficacy of its abstinence-only efforts as well. To the contrary, the actions of Drs. Crawford, Galson, and Hager are not exceptions; the Bush administration has actively suppressed and distorted information about the success of its abstinence and sex education programs.

First, the suppression.

In 2003, the Centers for Disease Control and Prevention (CDC) discontinued "Programs That Work," a flagship project that identified sex education programs that scientific studies have found to be effective.[45] According to a source inside CDC, a directive from "the White House" by way of the Department of Health and Human Services forced the agency to discontinue the project. All five of the initiatives identified as "Programs That Work" in 2002—their final year—involved comprehensive sex education for teenagers; none were abstinence-only programs. Not only did CDC end the project at the behest of Bush administration officials, it also removed all information about effective efforts from its government website.

This incident was not an anomaly.

One high-ranking scientist who worked at CDC from 2000 to 2005 offers a similar account. He told me that one of his department's major efforts was to publish an updated document entitled the "Compendium of HIV Prevention Interventions with Evidence of Effectiveness." This effort was begun during the Clinton administration as a focus of the so-called HIV/AIDS Prevention Research Synthesis Project. It is, in scope, reminiscent of the CDC's "Programs That Work" effort for sex education, only on a larger scale and with an arguably far greater effect on public health.[46]

To compile the compendium, a small, dedicated staff winnowed through the voluminous scientific literature on HIV/AIDS and community health initiatives to identify randomized control trials lasting six months or longer that showed positive effects. In other words, this CDC program was trying to use a sophisticated, relatively objective methodology to build a road map of scientifically based interventions that have proven effective in fighting the spread of AIDS.

This former CDC official, who asked not to be named, says the efforts to create an updated version of the compendium were repeatedly suppressed by the Bush administration at the highest levels, with the decision coming out of CDC director Julie Gerberding's office after consultations with her higher-ups at the Department of Health and Human Services. Presumably, he says, these officials were acting on either direct or implicit orders from the White House.

He says his group uncovered dozens of interventions that community-based health organizations need to know about. But during his tenure, his research group was unable to get its findings published by the government. As of this writing, the CDC group is making arrangements to have the compendium published by a peer-reviewed scientific journal so as to disseminate the vital federal research that the Bush administration has so far suppressed. U.S. public health, as this former CDC official puts it, is "unquestionably being put at risk by the Bush administration's policy in this case."

While the Bush administration has been unwilling to release the compendium, the former official says his group was ordered repeatedly to search for information that might cause political embarrassment to the administration. Several years ago, for instance, he says, the radio commentator Rush Limbaugh publicized the fact that a CDC website about the safe use of condoms included a list of possible non-petroleum-based lubricants for condoms including "grape jelly." Limbaugh exclaimed repeatedly on his show that "the government is teaching your daughter to have sex with grape jelly!" According to this source, Limbaugh's on-air statements resulted in "thousands of hours of reviews of government literature" in search of items that might cause similar embarrassment or derision. Internally, researchers at CDC have come to call such ongoing efforts "grape jelly reviews." As he eloquently puts it, "It was terribly frustrating: The Bush administration is suppressing the publication of studies paid for by American taxpayers. Instead they are giving us stuff we know won't work. The thing about science is that you make a commitment to share your results no matter what. Even from failure we learn. But this fundamental lesson has been badly undermined in the current administration."

And then there is the distortion: as disheartening as it may be that the federal government has suppressed information about what works to reduce teen pregnancies and sexually transmitted diseases, perhaps even more troubling is the fact that the Bush administration has rigged the federal government's own performance criteria in an effort to obscure how ineffective its abstinence-only programs are.

A decade ago, Congress passed and President Clinton signed the Government Performance and Results Act.[47] The law, which had overwhelming and bipartisan support, requires agencies to establish "objective, quantifiable, and measurable" indicators to assess whether government programs are working. When it comes to abstinence-only programs, though, the Bush administration has changed the evaluation criteria so that the programs won't be tracked for whether they actually have an effect on teenage birthrates or the prevalence of sexually transmitted diseases. In place of established criteria, such as charting the birthrate of female program participants, the government now tracks only participants' program attendance and attitudes, measures that actually obscure the lack of efficacy of abstinence-only programs.[48]

Initial performance measures for the federal government's abstinence-only funding, as required by the Government Performance and Results Act, were issued in November 2000 by an agency called Special Projects of Regional and National Significance (SPRANS), which administers much of the federal government's funding in this area. Those first SPRANS performance measures for abstinence-only education required the government, among other things, to track "the rate of births to female program participants." A year later, however, the Department of Health and Human Services altered these performance measures.

According to Donna Hutton, project officer for the Maternal and Children Health Bureau, "After we had published the [performance measures] guidance, the administration reviewed it and decided there were going to be some changes made to it."[49] At the behest of the Bush administration the criteria were changed to include six newly revised measures in place of the existing ones: henceforth, according to the new criteria, the government would track the numbers of people enrolled in the abstinence-only programs; the proportion of adolescents who say they "understand that abstinence from sexual activity is the only certain way to avoid out-of-wedlock pregnancy and sexually transmitted disease"; the proportion of adolescents "who indicate they understand the social, psychological, and health gains to be realized by abstaining from premarital sexual activity"; the proportion of participants who say they have gained the "refusal or assertiveness skills necessary to resist sexual urges and advances"; the proportion of youth "who *commit* to abstain from sexual activity until marriage" (emphasis added); and finally, the proportion of participants "who *intend to* avoid situations and risks, such as drug use and alcohol consumption, which make them more vulnerable to sexual advances and urges" (emphasis added).

Under the auspices of Rep. Henry Waxman (D-CA), an investigation by the minority staff of the House Committee on Government Reform looked at this issue in detail. It concluded that "the performance measures for abstinence-only programs represent a new development in the politicization of science: the manipulation of evaluation criteria to make programs favored by the right wing appear to be based on scientific evidence, when they are not."

As Waxman rightly concludes: "Notably, the new measures only address the attitudes of teens at the close of the program. No reports or assessments of actual behavior such as sexual activity rates, health outcomes such as pregnancy rates or sexually transmitted disease rates, or participant satisfaction with the program are included in the six current performance measures."[50]

PUBLIC HEALTH MALPRACTICE

These actions of the Bush administration, which would be dishonest in almost any context, must be specifically considered in the context of the AIDS epidemic. Put simply, people are dying in greater numbers because of Bush administration policies.

Worldwide, some forty million people are living with AIDS. Millions die annually, and some five million are newly infected with the virus each year. In the face of what we know to be largely a preventable epidemic, surely the first priority of the U.S. government's effort in this area must be to use our best science to protect people; to fund a wide array of public health and education activities; and to monitor their effectiveness.

For all the Bush administration's hollow moralizing, it is important to remember that, as *The Economist* eloquently editorialized:

AIDS is no respecter of morals: it affects babies as they are born, children as they are orphaned, nurses as they are accidentally pricked by a dirty needle, patients of any kind as they receive a transfusion of contaminated blood. Indeed, it affects the entire society in which its victims live and die. It also affects the faithful wife of the unfaithful husband.[51]

Internationally, however, during the Bush administration at least one-third of all U.S. government funds spent to prevent AIDS worldwide have been restricted to abstinence education. As a result, according to an April 2006 General Accountability Office study, the United States has weakened the global fight against AIDS. According to the report this requirement has meant that, in order to receive any aid at all, officials in some countries have had to reduce spending on programs to prevent the transmission of HIV from women to their newborn babies, as well as other prevention strategies stressing condom use.[52]

At home and abroad, when it comes to AIDS, it has been established beyond doubt that the best worldwide defense against its transmission is the use of latex condoms. And yet, in keeping with the Bush administration's abstinence-only policies, vital factual information about how effective condoms are in preventing the spread of AIDS has been removed from the CDC's website. Instead, the administration has mandated that the agency disseminate scientifically unfounded doubt about the efficacy of condoms in preventing the spread of HIV/AIDS.

Until October 2002, a fact sheet on the CDC website included information on proper condom use, the effectiveness of different types of condoms, and studies showing that condom education does not promote sexual activity. This information has been replaced with a document that emphasizes condom failure rates and the effectiveness of abstinence.[53]

Consider the public health implications of the message provided by the federal government before the Bush administration. The CDC fact sheet formerly read:

> Studies have shown that latex condoms are highly effective in preventing HIV transmission when used consistently and correctly. . . . The studies found that even with repeated sexual contact, 98–100 percent of those people who used latex condoms correctly and consistently did not become infected.

Now consider the message presented by the Bush administration. Today, the fact sheet reads:

> The surest way to avoid transmission of sexually transmitted disease [STD] is to abstain from sexual intercourse. . . . No protective method is 100 percent effective, and condom use cannot guarantee absolute protection against any STD.

When a source inside the CDC questioned the changes, she was told that they were directed by Bush administration officials at the Department of Health and Human Services.[54]

Given these kinds of actions, it is little wonder that so many medical professionals are outraged. "Public health malpractice is what the U.S. government is practicing," writes Thomas J. Coates, a professor of infectious diseases at UCLA Medical School. What else can you call it, Coates asks, when the government prescribes treatments known to be ineffective—such as abstinence pledges—and blocks information about the only effective tools we have—like condoms—to fight the spread of AIDS? As Coates rightly admonishes, "Public health requires the same adherence to scientific evidence as does clinical medicine."[55]

Among those most dismayed by Bush administration policies are medical specialists who continue to work in the federal government. Interviews with several current and recently departed staff members from the Centers from Disease Control, for example, present a disturbing picture of unprecedented interference by the Bush administration into the research and outreach activities of the agency. According to Margaret Scarlett, a former CDC staff member who served in the agency for fifteen years, most recently in the Office of HIV/AIDS policy, "The current administration has instituted an unheard-of level of micromanagement into the programmatic and scientific activities of CDC. We're seeing a clear substitution of ideology and an ideological bent for science, and it is causing many committed scientists to leave the agency."[56]

In just one example of politically motivated edicts at CDC, the Bush administration has decreed that any AIDS-fighting group in the United States that accepts federal money must include information on the lack of effectiveness of condom use in the content it produces. "The focus on everything has to be abstinence," said a longtime CDC scientist who asked not to be identified. "The language has to be scrutinized and approved at three thousand levels. The general sense is that propaganda has taken precedence over science."

One source, recently departed from a top-ranking position at CDC, recounts that, on at least one occasion, the administration required even top staff scientists at the agency to attend a daylong session purportedly devoted to the "science of abstinence." As this source puts it, "Out of the entire session, conducted by a nonscientist, the only thing resembling science was one study reportedly in progress and another not even begun." Despite the absence of supporting data, this source and others contend, CDC scientists were regularly reminded to push the administration's abstinence stance. As he puts it, "The effect was very chilling."[57]

Morale has reportedly plummeted at the CDC's Atlanta-based headquarters. For instance, in 2005 the *Washington Post* estimated that between retirements and widespread discontent, some forty CDC top managers—career professionals—had recently left the agency or were about to do so.[58] As Felicia Stewart, deputy assistant secretary of population affairs under President Clinton, noted, it will take federal agencies a long while to recover from the current loss of talent and expertise. And given the political climate and dissension, she says, "bright graduate students aren't going to be attracted to public-health areas. . . . They will see the controversy and say, I think I'll go into X-rays."[59]

John Santelli worked for CDC for thirteen years in the prevention of sexually transmitted diseases, until resigning in 2005. He put it this way: "You want an environment of open inquiry, but you see policy driven more by ideology than science."[60]

5

Clear Skies? Healthy Forests?

Understanding Bush's Real Environmental Policy

> Tinkering with scientific information, either striking it from reports or altering it, is becoming a pattern of behavior. It represents the politicizing of a scientific process, which at once manifests a disdain for professional scientists working for our government and a willingness to be less than candid with the American people.
>
> ROGER G. KENNEDY, former director of the National Park Service,
> *Los Angeles Times,* June 26, 2003

To understand the environmental policies of the Bush administration, it helps to consider a few things about the energy industry, particularly the companies that run the nation's gas-, oil-, and coal-fired electric power plants. No group is closer to the Bush administration philosophically, politically, or financially.

Philosophically speaking, the executives who control the nation's power plants tend to see their industries, quite literally, as the "turbines" that make the nation's economic growth possible. These executives also tend to be averse to any outside restrictions; they see their vital role as hampered by governmental regulation, especially environmental laws.

As former "oilmen" themselves, President George W. Bush and Vice President Dick Cheney thoroughly understand and share the views of these power company executives, and this perspective permeates the Bush administration. Michael O. Leavitt, now secretary of the Department of Health and Human Services, captured the sentiment clearly in an interview in 2004 while serving as head of the Environmental Protection Agency. "There is no environmental progress without economic prosperity. Once our competitiveness erodes, our capacity to make environmental gains is gone," Leavitt said. "There is nothing that promotes pollution like poverty."[1]

No sooner had the Bush administration come to power, in fact, than it began to flesh out a philosophical standpoint that treats environmental concerns as a luxury tied to economic growth. The perspective is exceptionally clear, for instance, in the Bush administration's National Energy Policy published in 2001.[2] Among the many priorities listed, the administration set out to remove or reduce wilderness and wildlife protections because of the perceived need to open up more public land to oil and gas exploration. The administration also explicitly sought to relax provisions in the decades-old Clean Air Act, replacing them with a market-based system favored by power plant owners in which companies buy, sell, and trade pollution rights.

Pollution is an important consideration for the nation's electric utility companies. Not only do the utilities tend to oppose regulation, but they are also among the nation's biggest polluters. As a group, power plants are the single largest industrial source of some of the worst kinds of air pollution. They produce more than two-thirds of the nation's annual emissions of sulfur dioxide, for instance, more than one-quarter of the nitrogen oxides, and one-third of all mercury emissions.[3]

These millions of tons of pollutants pumped into the air annually take a toll on the nation's health. The fine-particle pollution from power plants alone contributes to the deaths of an estimated thirty thousand Americans each year, according to one commonly cited estimate.[4] And, as we will discuss shortly, the health effects from mercury—which accumulates in the food chain—are substantial.

There is also something else important to note about air pollution from the nation's power plants: the dirtiest plants are highly concentrated among a surprisingly few energy companies. As documented in great detail by Eric Schaeffer, a former top EPA enforcement official, in a report entitled *America's Dirtiest Power Plants: Plugged into the Bush Administration*, 43 percent of all the sulfur dioxide released into the air by the entire power industry comes from just fifty of the nation's top sulfur dioxide emitters.[5]

To complete the picture, Schaeffer's 2004 report documents that the nation's biggest, most polluting, most vociferously antiregulation companies were also the largest single group of contributors to George W.

Bush in both the 2000 and 2004 elections. Since 1999, the thirty utility companies that own the nation's most polluting plants have poured some $6.6 million into the coffers of the Bush presidential campaigns and the Republican National Committee. Put another way, there were more executives from energy than from any other industry group among Mr. Bush's most elite fund-raisers, called "Pioneers," each of whom generated more than $100,000 in donations.[6]

After raising millions of dollars to elect George W. Bush, many of the biggest utility donors were granted extraordinary access to his administration. They were invited to join the transition team and to serve on the committees that nominated officials to serve in the new administration. Many of them were thus able to help handpick the government officials who would be given senior positions in charge of formulating or enforcing air pollution policies.

Schaeffer's careful research shows that the thirty big power plant companies hired at least fourteen lobbying firms that met with Vice President Cheney's national energy task force at least seventeen times to help formulate the country's energy and pollution policies.[7] Also at many of the meetings was Thomas Kuhn, a Bush classmate at Yale and now the president of the Edison Electric Institute, the trade association for most coal-fired electric utility corporations (and himself a Bush "Pioneer" fund-raiser for both 2000 and 2004).

Although the Bush administration eventually went all the way to the U.S. Supreme Court to withhold the details of the energy task force meetings from the American public, we know that this group's recommendations led directly to a strategy to change the nation's air pollution laws. The bottom line was this: the power plants didn't want to be hampered by environmental regulations, and the Bush administration—for philosophical, political, *and* financial reasons—didn't want them to be either.

In particular, for the electric utilities, one issue towered above all others when the Bush administration first came into office. Over the course of the 1980s and 1990s, the nation's electric power plant owners were starting to feel the pinch of the Clean Air Act. One of its important provisions, called New Source Review, required power plants to make use of less-polluting technology when they modernized. This environmentally and economically smart legislation was added to the Clean Air Act in 1977.[8] It didn't mandate costly changes immediately from industry; rather, it gradually forced the industry to take advantage of the environmentally best technology available as it spent money for plant upgrades. As Bruce C. Buckheit, then director of Air Enforcement at EPA put it, through the New Source Review provisions, "On sulfur dioxide alone we expected to get several million tons per year out of the atmosphere."[9]

When the time came to modernize, however, many power plant owners routinely disobeyed the law. Presumably figuring that the government wouldn't enforce its provisions, these companies modernized without adding the required pollution controls. This illegal activity may have saved the power plants money, but it exacted a huge toll on the nation's health and air quality. Sylvia Lowrance, EPA's top official for enforcement and compliance from 1996 to 2002, called the behavior of the power plant owners "the most significant noncompliance pattern EPA had ever found."[10]

Recognizing that the federal government had a huge enforcement issue on its hands, the Environmental Protection Agency began in 1997, during the Clinton administration, to investigate these power plants for noncompliance with the nation's environmental laws. In 1999, on behalf of EPA, the U.S. Justice Department sued nine utility companies, charging that they had expanded fifty-one older plants without adding the required controls. These power plants, the government alleged, had been illegally releasing enormous quantities of pollution, in some cases for twenty years or more. Taken together, the companies named in the suits emitted more than 2 million tons of sulfur dioxide and 660,000 tons of nitrogen oxides every year.[11]

Environmentally and economically, the stakes of the federal government's enforcement lawsuits were high. And a small but powerful group of electric utility companies was especially unhappy and motivated to seek whatever redress they could in a new federal administration.

Soon after coming to office, top Bush administration officials devised a multipronged strategy to benefit the electric utility companies. One piece of the strategy involved the courts. The Bush administration ordered the Justice Department to review the EPA enforcement cases against the noncompliant electric utility companies to see whether they might be dropped. But, much to the utilities' chagrin, in January 2002, the Justice Department ruled that the lawsuits were brought on legitimate grounds.

Especially in light of the ruling, the Bush administration then began to emphasize the most visible of its strategies to help the electric utilities: its legislative plan. On February 14, 2002, President Bush unveiled his Clear Skies Initiative. The president declared that his proposed legislation "set tough new standards to dramatically reduce the three most significant forms of pollution from power plants—sulfur dioxide, nitrogen oxide and mercury."[12] But, in fact, the Bush plan was a cynically titled gift to the energy industry. "Clear Skies" proposed to replace Clean Air Act regulations with a cap-and-trade market system that would allow 50 percent more sulfur dioxide, nearly 40 percent more nitrogen oxides, and three times as much mercury than the Clean Air Act allowed if it were rigorously enforced. The Bush administration's Clear Skies Initiative also proposed to delay cleaning up this pollution by as much as a decade beyond current law. As a result, residents of heavily polluted areas would have to wait years longer for reductions in pollutants than under the existing Clean Air Act.[13]

Even with its Madison Avenue name and a Republican-dominated U.S. Congress, Clear Skies was a tough sell. It didn't help that, around the time of the initiative's announcement, Eric Schaeffer left his top position in EPA enforcement in protest and appeared on television, explaining, "We can do better under current law than what they're putting on the table."[14]

But, even as Clear Skies met with opposition in Congress, the Bush administration had its most effective strategy already at work: the quiet subversion of the nation's environmental laws through regulatory changes and bureaucratic maneuvers.

"One key element of the strategy was putting the right people in under-the-radar positions," the reporter Bruce Barcott explained in detail in the *New York Times Sunday Magazine*. "The Bush administration appointed officials who came directly from industry into these lower rungs of power—deputy secretaries and assistant administrators. These second-tier appointees knew exactly which rules and regulations to change because they had been trying to change them, on behalf of their industries, for years."[15]

MEET JEFFREY HOLMSTEAD

In the area of federal air pollution regulations, no appointment has been more important to the Bush administration than that of Jeffrey R. Holmstead, EPA's assistant administrator for Air and Radiation. Holmstead, who left the post in August 2005, was a consummate insider. Throughout his career, he worked on behalf of corporate clients to scale back and minimize the effects of environmental regulation on business. He served as an associate White House counsel in the administration of George H. W. Bush, and he spent the years of the Clinton administration as a partner in the environmental department of the Washington DC–based law firm Latham and Watkins—a firm that represented several electric utilities trying to fight air pollution regulations.[16]

Holmstead played an important role for the Bush administration when, in 2003, a group of four senators—Thomas Carper (D-DE), Judd Gregg (R-NH), Lamar Alexander (R-TN), and Lincoln Chafee (R-RI)— proposed an alternative to the president's Clear Skies Act. The so-called Carper amendment sought to control carbon dioxide in addition to sulfur dioxide, nitrogen oxides, and mercury.[17] Although EPA evaluated this proposal, the agency withheld most of the results from the senators for several months after they were requested. Before EPA officials finally provided the material to the senators, a copy of a briefing based on the study was leaked to the *Washington Post*. According to the briefing, EPA scientists had concluded that the so-called Carper amendment would cut the three pollutants earlier and in larger quantity than the Clear Skies Act, resulting in 17,800 fewer expected deaths by 2020. EPA scientists also determined that the senators' proposal would reduce carbon dioxide emissions at "negligible" cost to industry.[18]

The suppression of research on air pollution is of serious concern because of its enormous impact on public health. The Clean Air Act, which passed during the Nixon administration and was strengthened in 1990 during the first Bush administration, has improved air quality and saved American lives. According to an EPA analysis of the period up to 1990, if the Clean Air Act had not been enacted,

an additional 205,000 Americans would have died prematurely and millions more would have suffered illnesses ranging from mild respiratory symptoms to heart disease, chronic bronchitis, asthma attacks, and other severe respiratory problems. In addition, the lack of the Clean Air Act controls on the use of leaded gasoline would have resulted in major increases in child IQ loss and adult hypertension, heart disease and stroke.[19]

As reported in the *New York Times,* EPA staff members stated that, in a May 2003 meeting with Holmstead, they discussed the unreleased report indicating the advantages of the Carper amendment. At that meeting, according to these EPA staffers, Holmstead wondered out loud, "How can we justify Clear Skies if this gets out?" When questioned about the matter by reporters, however, Holmstead stated that he did not "recall making any specific remarks at the meeting."[20]

Ultimately, in March 2005, President Bush's Clear Skies plan stalled in committee and never reached the Senate floor. But, despite the defeat for the administration, Holmstead was able to do arguably more for the electric utilities than even the Clear Skies initiative would have. The Bush administration realized that it could subvert the intent of New Source Review (NSR) provisions by changing the government's technical definition of where to draw the line between routine plant maintenance and the significant overhauls that would trigger NSR provisions. Jeffrey Holmstead, in his under-the-radar position, was in a perfect position to do something about it.

At about the same time that the Clear Skies proposal was announced, Holmstead asked Sylvia Lowrance, then EPA's deputy assistant administrator for enforcement, to suggest a financial threshold—a percentage of the total value of each generator that a utility would be permitted to spend on renovations and still define them as routine. Lowrance, a twenty-four-year veteran of the agency, had officials in her office study years of data, looking at figures that came from actual power plants. On June 3, 2002, she wrote a memo to Holmstead (later leaked to reporters) indicating that her office thought 0.75 percent was a reasonable figure. In other words, EPA analysts in Lowrance's office determined that if the total value of a generating unit was $1 billion, a power company should be able to legitimately spend up to $7.5 million without being required to install new pollution controls.

In August 2003, Holmstead unveiled the EPA's finalized rule on routine maintenance. The new formula did not adopt the threshold suggested by Lowrance and her team of EPA analysts, or anything close. Instead, under the Bush administration's plan, utilities would be allowed to spend *up to 20 percent* of a generating unit's replacement costs per year without tripping the NSR threshold.

As Barcott reported in the *New York Times Sunday Magazine,* Frank O'Donnell, the executive director of the nonprofit Clean Air Trust, called the Bush threshold "a moron test" for power companies: "It's such a huge loophole," O'Donnell said, "that only a moron would trip over it and become subject to NSR requirements." Eric Schaeffer, the former EPA enforcement official, stated: "Five percent would have been too high, but 20? I don't think the industry expected that in its wildest dreams." The American Lung Association, in a report issued with a coalition of environmental groups, called the rule changes on New Source Review "the most harmful and unlawful air pollution initiative ever undertaken by the federal government."[21]

The bureaucratic undermining of the New Source Review legislation clearly illustrates a strategy by the Bush administration to benefit industry by manipulating the government's handling of technical information and subverting the intent of a provision of federal law. The same kinds of tactics have been used repeatedly by the administration. To more fully appreciate the strategy, let's consider the way scientific and technical information was handled by Holmstead and the Bush administration to bypass rules governing air emissions of mercury.

MERCURY POLLUTION: "TRADING IN" THE NATION'S HEALTH

First, some background is in order. Mercury is a neurotoxin that can cause brain damage and harm reproduction in women and wildlife. It is retained in body tissue and accumulates in the food chain. Coal-fired power plants are the nation's largest source of mercury air emissions, emitting about 48 tons annually.[22] Under the Clinton administration a set of rules—the so-called Maximum Achievable Control Technology (MACT), required under the Clean Air Act—mandated reducing these emissions by as much as 90 percent by 2008. MACT offered a great environmental benefit, but it was also a costly requirement for the power plants to meet. As soon as Bush administration officials came to power, they sought a means to avoid regulating mercury emissions by coal-fired power plants.[23]

In pursuit of this goal, senior Bush officials began by suppressing government information about mercury contained in an EPA report on children's health and the environment. As the EPA readied the report for completion in May 2002, the White House Office of Management and Budget and the Office of Science and Technology Policy (OSTP) requested a review of the document. This turned out to be a ploy for shelving the report. In February 2003, after nine months of "review" by the White House, a frustrated EPA official leaked the draft report to the *Wall Street Journal,* including its finding that 8 percent of U.S. women between the ages of sixteen and forty-nine have mercury levels in the blood that could lead to reduced IQ and motor skills in their offspring.[24]

The finding provided strong evidence in direct opposition to the administration's desired policy of reducing regulation on coal-fired power plants, which was undoubtedly the reason for the lengthy suppression by the White House. On February 24, 2003, just days after the leak, the Bush administration finally released the EPA report on mercury to the public.[25] As in similar cases involving Bush administration officials, the troubling timing suggested that the report might never have surfaced at all if it had not been leaked to the press.

In March 2004, the Bush administration proposed a new regulation for coal-fired power plants. These rules involved a so-called cap-and-trade system favored by industry and by the Bush administration, in which companies can buy, sell, and trade pollution rights to achieve an overall industry target. The Bush administration's plan proposed to reduce mercury emissions by 30 percent over the next fifteen years—instead of reducing them by 90 percent by 2008.[26] The twenty-seven-member Children's Health Protection Advisory Committee—a government advisory group that includes health experts from state and federal agencies, environmental groups, universities, and corporations such as Bayer, BP, Monsanto, and Procter and Gamble—urged EPA administrator Mike Leavitt to reconsider the plan.[27]

As many experts inside and outside of the government pointed out, the deadly problem with such an approach for a toxin like mercury is that it can create toxic "hot spots" in some communities near mercury polluters that choose to buy pollution rights. According to the Natural Resources Defense Council, for instance, the Bush administration's mercury plan would dramatically increase mercury pollution in California, Colorado, and New Hampshire. William Becker, director of the bipartisan State and Territorial Air Pollution Program Administrators, did not mince words about the plan. He called it "unconscionable" for the Bush administration to allow power companies to trade in a powerful neurotoxin. "It is unprecedented and illegal," Becker said.[28]

Drawing upon interviews with no fewer than five current career employees at EPA, reporters at the *Los Angeles Times* exposed in detail the process that led to the proposed mercury regulations, documenting how Bush administration political appointees at EPA bypassed agency professional and scientific staff in crafting the proposed new rules.[29] Bruce Buckheit, who had retired in December 2003 as director of EPA's Air Enforcement Division after serving in major federal environmental posts for two decades, says that his enforcement division was not even allowed to review the mercury regulations before their release: "The new mercury rules were hatched at the White House. The Environmental Protection Agency's experts were simply not consulted at all."[30]

As the *Los Angeles Times* reported, the topic of the new Bush administration mercury rules was discussed in the spring of 2004 at an EPA staff meeting presided over by Holmstead. According to reports from five separate staff members, EPA scientists had expected to discuss plans to carry out comparative studies of proposals to reduce mercury emissions. The studies, which had been requested by the Children's Health Protection Advisory Committee, would examine the effects of mercury regulation on energy markets, electricity prices, and public health. This type of analysis, generated through EPA computer models, typically becomes the basis upon which agency officials and outsiders weigh alternative policy options.

At this meeting, however, William Wehrum, a senior adviser to Holmstead, who like his boss had represented industry clients at the law firm Latham and Watkins before joining the Bush administration, told the dozen staffers at the meeting that comparative studies would be postponed indefinitely. "I was floored," said one participant, who has served several administrations. "We pointed out that the studies were required . . . that the data runs were promised to a federal advisory committee." But neither Holmstead nor Wehrum, who has since replaced Holmstead as assistant administrator for Air and Radiation, responded to such expressions of concern, participants said. As one recalled: "There was an awkward silence."[31]

After the meeting, two EPA staff members say that they personally complained to Holmstead that comparative scientific studies of the effects of the proposed rules were required by EPA procedure. But these sources contend Holmstead told them that such studies would not be conducted, partly because of "White House concern."[32]

In March 2005, the Bush administration released the final version of its Clean Air Mercury Rule, with a cap-and-trade system that will reduce mercury emissions less and far more slowly than the Clean Air Act had mandated.[33] The new rule gives industry the reprieve it had sought. In fact, the rule's promulgation was largely an industry production from start to finish. As noted in chapter 1, in its proposed form, the EPA rule's preamble was even discovered to contain no fewer than twelve paragraphs lifted, sometimes verbatim, from a legal document prepared by industry lawyers at Latham and Watkins—where Holmstead and Wehrum worked before joining the Bush administration.[34]

Outraged public health and environmental advocates contend the new mercury rule violates the 1990 Clean Air Act, ignores the science on mercury hazards, and allows industry to pollute beyond the 2018 deadline. Eleven states have already sued the agency, challenging the rule.[35]

The states have a strong case. In the aftermath of this episode, two separate government reviews have criticized the Bush administration's procedures in the matter as badly flawed. In February 2005, a report released by the EPA inspector general concluded that processes used to promulgate the new mercury rule were "inconsistent with expected and past EPA practices, including a failure to fully assess the rule's impact on children's health."[36] A similar review of the episode by the Government Accountability Office (GAO), released in March 2005, criticized the process for its lack of "transparency" and concluded that EPA had failed to fully document the toxic impact of mercury on brain development, learning, and neurological function. The GAO urged that the problems be rectified before the EPA takes final action on the rule.[37]

The episode also left a demoralized collection of government scientists and staff members in its wake. Buckheit, who had resigned in December

2003 in protest of the Bush administration's lack of integrity in the policy process, says he cannot recall another instance when the agency's technical experts were so thoroughly shut out of the process in developing a major regulatory proposal. According to Buckheit, the incident is representative of "a degree of politicization of the work of the Environmental Protection Agency that goes beyond anything I have seen in my career in government."[38] Buckheit, who had served in major federal environmental posts for two decades, had come to feel that enforcement was stymied. "A political agenda is driving the agency's output, rather than analysis and science," he said.[39]

MANIPULATING THE SCIENTIFIC PROCESS FOR THE TIMBER INDUSTRY

As the EPA's top air pollution regulator, Jeffrey Holmstead used many of the same tactics to weaken environmental regulations for other industries besides the electric utilities. A good example can be seen in his intervention in setting EPA's "safe" levels of formaldehyde, a chemical used widely in the manufacture of building materials and household products. It is also released when wood, tobacco, and other organic substances burn. Formaldehyde is known to cause nausea and eye, throat, and skin irritation. Recent studies by the National Cancer Institute and the National Institute of Occupational Safety and Health also link formaldehyde exposure to leukemia in humans.[40] But with Holmstead's intervention, EPA disregarded these studies to create a new air pollution regulation, relying instead on a risk assessment generated by an organization funded by the chemical industry. The new regulation is about ten thousand times weaker than the level previously used by the EPA in setting standards for formaldehyde exposure.[41]

The formaldehyde story, like so many others, represents a small piece of a much bigger picture. Across the board, and at a number of different federal agencies, the Bush administration has made a point of supporting the timber industry. Just as the administration has sought to undermine air pollution laws that it sees as costly restrictions on the electric power industry, Bush officials have tended to see restrictions on logging on public lands as a needless restriction on economic growth.

With its Clear Skies Initiative, the Bush administration sought to ease pollution restrictions. Similarly, its so-called Healthy Forests plan sought to open public lands to more logging. Consider just one of numerous interventions along these lines. Forest management itself has been another area of particular concern to the Bush administration, which in 2003 created a "review team" made up predominantly of nonscientists who proceeded to overrule the Sierra Nevada Framework, a $12-million science-based plan for managing old-growth forest habitat and reducing the risk of fire in eleven national forests. This plan, adopted by the Clinton administration after nine years of research by more than one hundred scientists from the Forest Service and academia, had been regarded by the experts who reviewed it as an exemplary use of credible science in forest policy.[42]

The Bush administration's proposed changes to the plan include harvesting more of the largest trees, which may double or triple harvest levels over the first ten years of the plan.[43] Other changes call for relaxing restrictions on cattle grazing in some areas where the original plan significantly reduced grazing because of the potentially critical impact on sensitive species.

Forest Service officials justified these changes in part by stating that the original plan relied too much on prescribed burning and would fail to "effectively protect the general forest areas from fire."[44] Indeed, ecologically sustainable thinning that minimizes risks to threatened and endangered species may also be an appropriate tool for reducing risk of catastrophic fire in these forests.[45] Contrary to Forest Service claims that their recommendations are based on "new information and findings," however, the revisions designed to substantially increase timber harvests reflect a policy choice that prioritizes fire management (and profit) over species protection, and lack a foundation in the best available science.[46] In fact, a scientific review panel put together by the Forest Service found that the revisions failed to consider key scientific information regarding fire, impacts on forest health, and endangered species.[47]

MEET STEPHEN GRILES

As we have seen at EPA and elsewhere, the Bush administration has made a practice of installing industry advocates in key regulatory and enforcement positions in the federal government. Perhaps nowhere has the practice had such a devastating impact on the environment as at the U.S. Department of the Interior. In one such tale of the manipulation of scientific data, J. Stephen Griles, a deputy secretary at the Department of the Interior, authorized the distortion of the government's environmental reports to back environmentally damaging coal mining techniques.

Over the past decade, the practice of mountaintop removal strip mining has been widely used to extract coal in central Appalachia. In this process, huge machines remove the tops of mountain ridges to expose coal seams; millions of tons of waste rock and dirt are then dumped into nearby hollows, burying mountain headwater streams under enormous "valley fills." As part of a 1998 court settlement, the federal government agreed to produce an Environmental Impact Statement (EIS) analyzing the effects of this practice and finding ways to limit the environmental damage caused, especially to streams in the region.[48]

According to the National Environmental Protection Act (NEPA) of 1969, an explicit purpose of an EIS is to list alternative possibilities, with a specific technical assessment of the environmental implications of the practices being reviewed.[49] However, internal government documents obtained under the Freedom of Information Act reveal that Griles, a former lobbyist for the National Mining Association,[50] instructed agency scientists and staff to undermine some $8 million worth of scientific studies conducted by five separate federal and state agencies over four years in preparation of the EIS on mountaintop removal mining required by the 1998 settlement. [51]

Under Griles's direction, agencies were told to drop consideration of any options for more environmentally benign alternatives to current practices, despite overwhelming scientific evidence of environmental destruction from the technique.[52] In addition, technical language required by NEPA to rate environmental impacts on a scale from "not significant" to "severe" was edited to remove the classifications of "very significant" and "severe."[53]

A now-public memo from Griles to the White House Council on Environmental Quality and other federal agencies involved in the EIS shows that Griles directed that a new draft EIS should "focus on centralizing and streamlining coal-mining permitting" instead of studying ways to limit the environmental damage caused by mountaintop removal and valley fills.[54]

To appreciate the scale of the environmental consequences of Griles's ruling, consider that, for the past several years, scientists working for various federal agencies have documented a wide range of enormously destructive environmental impacts from this mining technique. Over 7 percent of Appalachian forests have been cut down, and more than twelve hundred miles of streams across the region have been buried or polluted by valley fills, between 1985 and 2001 in the course of mountaintop removal mining.[55] According to the federal government's scientific analysis, mountaintop removal mining, if it continues unabated, will cause a projected loss of over 1.4 million acres—an area the size of Delaware—by the end of the next decade with a concomitant severe impact on fish, wildlife, and bird species.[56]

While the EIS produced by the Bush administration includes analysis documenting this destruction, Griles's ruling effectively distorted and undermined the report's overwhelmingly negative findings. Most importantly, the ruling violated a central tenet of an EIS by offering no proposed alternatives to mitigate the worst environmental consequences of mountaintop removal mining.

As noted, the Bush administration team ordered scientists to strip away technical language rating the environmental impacts as "very significant" or "severe." In addition, the steering committee led by Griles initially removed an entire economic analysis prepared by an independent contractor that showed that limits on the size of individual valley fills would have virtually no negative economic impacts on the region's electric costs. The steering committee discredited the study's methodology. But a revised analysis, which took into account the comments and concerns of dozens of coal industry officials, still found that the economic costs of limiting the size of valley fills would have a negligible effect on the price of coal.[57]

"We were flabbergasted and outraged," says one high-ranking staff scientist at the U.S. Fish and Wildlife Service who had worked extensively on the preparation of the technical analysis for the environmental impact statement. This official, whose name is withheld on request, explains that the Bush administration "steering committee" of the interagency EIS process called a meeting in October 2001 at which agency scientists and administrators were told that the draft EIS "was going to be taken in a different direction." Rather than present alternatives to reduce the environmental harm caused by mountaintop removal mining and valley fills, the team was directed by the steering committee to develop more efficient procedures to issue permits for mountaintop removal mining to make it easier for the practice to continue unabated.[58]

Cindy Tibbot, a Fish and Wildlife Service biologist involved in the EIS process, was one of many agency scientists who expressed outrage about the plan, stating in an internal memo, "It's hard to stay quiet about this when I really believe we're doing the public and the heart of the Clean Water Act a great disservice." As Tibbot put it, the only alternatives Griles's proposed EIS would offer would be "alternative locations to house the rubber stamp that issues the [mining] permits."[59]

Tibbot was not alone. An internal memo from U.S. Fish and Wildlife staff reviewing the draft EIS before its release assessed the situation this way:

> The EIS technical studies carried out by the agencies—at considerable taxpayer expense—have documented adverse impacts to aquatic and terrestrial ecosystems, yet the proposed alternatives presented offer no substantive means of addressing these impacts. The alternatives and actions, as currently written, belie four years of work and the accumulated evidence of environmental harms, and would substitute permit process tinkering for meaningful and measurable change. Publication of a draft EIS with this approach, especially when the public has seen earlier drafts, will further damage the credibility of the agencies involved.[60]

Recently obtained documents reveal that staff members at other agencies involved in the EIS process were equally concerned with the administration's approach to the EIS. Ray George, an EPA official from West Virginia's Region 3, complained that his agency's "science findings are not reflected in [the draft EIS's] conclusions/recommendations."[61] Another EPA official, John Forren, underscored the severity of the problem. "It's one thing," he wrote, "to include such alternatives in the EIS and not choose one as a preferred alternative or not choose one as the selected action in the Record of Decision." It was quite another thing to offer no meaningful alternatives at all. Such a tactic "give[s] the appearance we're obscuring and de-emphasizing the [alternatives] that address directly environmental impacts" and could, Forren warned, leave the entire EIS process open to legal challenge and public outcry.[62]

"In this case, the administration eliminated all environmental protective alternatives from consideration," says Jim Hecker, environmental enforcement director at Trial Lawyers for Public Justice, who filed the Freedom of Information Act request for the internal documents in this case. As Hecker puts it, "The simple fact is: that is scientifically and intellectually dishonest."[63]

Many high-ranking government scientists are troubled by the close financial ties between the Bush administration and the energy industry as well as the apparent conflict of interest presented by J. Stephen Griles's close involvement in the EIS process. Aware of Griles's long-standing association with the mining industry, the U.S. Senate requested that he sign a "statement of disqualification" on August 1, 2001, in which he made a commitment to avoid issues affecting his former clients. Nonetheless, documents obtained under the Freedom of Information Act show that Griles met no fewer than twelve times with top Bush administration officials and coal industry representatives on the EIS and mountaintop removal mining matters between September and December 2001, precisely the time the team issued its directive to "change direction" on the EIS process.[64]

During the EIS official comment period, representatives from fifty environmental groups across the country wrote a letter charging that the draft EIS failed to comply with the National Environmental Protection Act: "We find the draft EIS's failure to provide an alternative proposal that would provide better regulation of mountaintop removal mining to protect the environment unacceptable and inappropriate."[65] Former Maryland state senator Gerald Winegrad, a vice president of the American Bird Conservancy and co-author of the letter, compared the potential for environmental destruction from mountaintop removal mining with the impacts of drilling for oil in the Arctic National Wildlife Refuge. Our political process cannot function, Winegrad says, without an honest scientific assessment of the problem. "But in this case," he says, "the EIS process has been usurped and its scientific underpinnings destroyed."[66]

6

When Good Science Is the Endangered Species

The members of our panel were told to either strip out our recommendations or see our report end up in a drawer.

ROBERT PAINE, ecologist at the University of Washington, April 2004

By this point, a few things should be clear about the Bush administration: it is driven by ideology and political payback to its core constituencies. Top administration officials often appear to place little
value on science as a tool to inform policymaking. And at the explicit direction of the White House, Bush appointees have repeatedly suppressed,
ignored, or even distorted facts inconvenient to predetermined policies.

It should also be clear that the Bush administration follows essentially
the same "playbook" across a range of scientific issues and at diverse federal agencies. Some observers even credit the administration's disciplined
politics-trumps-science approach to the political direction of a single so-
called architect: Karl Rove. One commentator, for instance, has likened
Rove to the "system coach" in team sports who, regardless of circum-
stance, follows the predetermined plays he or she has devised to ensure
victory.[1]

Given the Bush administration's well-known desire to tightly control
all information about its internal workings, it is difficult to establish the
precise chain of command that has yielded so consistent a pattern of scientific misconduct. Regardless, whether the cases derive from one particular White House mind or several, a general climate is communicated
from the highest levels that the administration has "made up its mind"
on many topics of national concern, no matter what the data might sug-

gest. This climate is, of course, anathema to the conduct of impartial scientific research.

A prime example is surely the Bush administration's evident view that industrial development in the United States is hampered by the protection of threatened and endangered species.

Of course, the administration is not alone in this view. Most Americans are familiar with stories in which a demonstrated threat to an endangered bird, fish, or small-mammal population has stymied development. By and large, the American people favor protecting the natural environment, yet it is possible to make a persuasive case that the protection of endangered species has in some respects gone too far and that the 1973 Endangered Species Act (ESA) ought to be reviewed and amended. The administration is, in fact, pushing to amend that act, but a frontal assault is not the preferred strategy in the Bush playbook. Rather, its modus operandi is to squelch findings and subvert existing laws that run counter to its goals.

Consider, first, the number of new species listed as threatened or endangered since 2001. According to one systematic review, the Bush administration has listed only twenty-five species since coming to office—all under court order. By contrast, the Clinton administration listed an average of sixty-five species *each year,* and Bush senior's administration listed an average of fifty-eight yearly.[2]

Of course, the listing of threatened and endangered species tells only a piece of the story. The budget the Bush administration has sent to Congress has proposed funding cuts each year for enforcing the Endangered Species Act, and, according to a wide array of scientists, government officials, and environmental groups, the administration has systematically sought to weaken other protections for the nation's most threatened animal species.[3] For instance, it has supported amendments pending before Congress that would make it harder to list threatened and endangered species by limiting the use of population modeling, the technique that offers the most credible way to assess the likelihood that a small population of a given species will survive in a given habitat.[4]

But perhaps most troubling has been the way in which the Bush administration has suppressed and even sought to distort its own agencies' scientific findings. These actions, which go well beyond a debate over the Endangered Species Act, represent a manipulation of the scientific underpinnings of the policymaking process itself. Concerns about this issue come not only from critics outside the government but from scientists within. As mentioned briefly earlier, a survey of some four hundred scientists in the U.S. Fish and Wildlife Service conducted by two nonprofit groups—the Public Employees for Environmental Responsibility and the Union of Concerned Scientists—asked a variety of questions about the politicization of science. The responses are eye-opening indeed.

Close to half the respondents whose work relates to scientific findings that form the basis for listing endangered species reported that they have been directed, "for non-scientific reasons, to refrain from making . . . findings that are protective of species." One in five agency scientists say they have been instructed to compromise their individual scientific integrity, responding affirmatively when asked if they had ever been "directed to inappropriately exclude or alter technical information from a scientific document."[5] As one U.S. Fish and Wildlife biologist told the *Los Angeles Times:* "For biologists who do endangered species analysis, my experience is that the majority of them are ordered to reverse their conclusions [if they favor listing]. There are other biologists who will do it if you won't."[6]

Little wonder that reversals of scientific conclusions led two members of Congress—Rep. Henry Waxman (D-CA), the ranking minority member of the House Committee on Government Reform, and Rep. Nick Rahall (D-WV), the ranking minority member of the House Committee on Resources—to send an angry letter to Secretary of the Interior Gale Norton. As the congressmen put it: "The picture that emerges is appalling. The Fish and Wildlife Service's credibility rests on its scientific integrity. If political agendas are allowed to overrule science, that credibility will be compromised."[7]

To what extent has that integrity been compromised at the U.S. Fish and Wildlife Service? The evidence paints a picture of a very troubled agency.

TROUT BULL

In 2004, U.S. Fish and Wildlife Service (FWS) officials censored an analysis of the economics of protecting the bull trout, a species in the Pacific

Northwest that has been listed under the Endangered Species Act since 1998. FWS published only an inflated assessment of the costs associated with protecting the species and deleted the report's section analyzing the economic benefits.[8]

This story begins with a 2003 court settlement in which the Fish and Wildlife Service agreed to develop a plan designating critical habitat in the Pacific Northwest for bull trout.[9] The settlement came after a local environmental group had sued the agency for failing to protect the fish. In conjunction with the settlement, the Fish and Wildlife Service contracted with Bioeconomics, Inc., of Missoula, Montana, to conduct a cost-benefit analysis of bull trout recovery in Oregon, Washington, Idaho, and Montana. The firm's peer-reviewed research determined that protecting the bull trout and its habitat in the Columbia and Klamath river basins would cost $230 million to $300 million over a decade; it derived these costs based on projected adverse effects upon hydropower, logging, and highway construction. Notably, however, the study also reported that $215 million in economic benefits would be associated with a restored bull trout fishery.[10]

When officials at the Fish and Wildlife Service released the analysis, however, they deleted the fifty-five pages of the report that analyzed the economic benefits of bull trout recovery.[11]

An exaggerated cost analysis and a deleted benefits analysis essentially gave FWS the economic justification, under the Endangered Species Act, to disregard scientific information on designating critical habitats for the endangered bull trout.[12] But the censorship spurred an anonymous FWS employee to leak the deleted chapter to Alliance for the Wild Rockies, a Montana-based environmental group, which then passed it to the *Missoulian,* a Montana daily newspaper. Upon questioning from the press, Diane Katzenberger, an information officer in the FWS Denver regional office, said that the censorship did not occur in either the Denver or Portland regional FWS offices but rather "was a policy decision made at the Washington level."[13]

Chris Nolin, chief of the division of conservation and classification in the FWS Washington office, told the press that the benefits analysis was cut because its methodology was discouraged by the Office of Management and Budget.[14] However, the Bush administration has released numerous benefits analyses using the same methodology. In February

2003, for instance, the Environmental Protection Agency used these methods to estimate that $113 billion in economic benefits over ten years would result from implementing the administration's 2003 Clear Skies Initiative.[15]

According to Michael Garrity, executive director of Alliance for the Wild Rockies, the benefits estimate is based largely on solid economic projections of income from sport fishing. His group has publicly asked FWS to release the full economic analysis. As of this writing, it is not clear whether FWS will use the truncated analysis released to date to trump scientific considerations, but the stage is clearly set for such an outcome.[16]

OPEN SEASON ON TRUMPETER SWANS

Bull trout are hardly the only species whose protection is threatened by Bush administration policies. According to documents released through a Freedom of Information Act request by the watchdog group Public Employees for Environmental Responsibility, the former director of the Fish and Wildlife Service, Steven A. Williams, decided not to list the rare trumpeter swan *(Cygnus buccinator)* as endangered based on two documents: a scientifically flawed non-peer-reviewed report and a seriously misrepresented peer-reviewed study.[17] Williams overruled the unanimous recommendation of his own scientific review panel and refused to release that panel's report.

Conservationists had petitioned Williams to list the tristate trumpeter swans (so called because they breed in the Rocky Mountain states of Montana, Wyoming, and Idaho) as threatened or endangered under the Endangered Species Act. The tristate Rocky Mountain trumpeter swans constitute the only breeding population that survives in the lower forty-eight states, where this species was once common. Migrating tristate trumpeters, which resemble the more plentiful tundra swans, winter in Utah, and some number are virtually always killed during the annual tundra swan hunt there. Environmentalists and ornithologists had sought since 2000 to protect the tristate Rocky Mountain trumpeters—North America's largest waterfowl—under the Endangered Species Act.[18] If trumpeter swans were designated as a threatened species, however, FWS would be forced to halt the popular hunting season of tundra swans in Utah. In response to environmentalists' prodding, FWS produced a controversial internal document for agency review that argues the Rocky Mountain trumpeter swans do not constitute what is called a "distinct population segment" but are actually part of a much larger population of trumpeter swans in Canada and Alaska.[19] James Dubovsky and John Cornely, the two scientists who wrote the report, never submitted it for peer review, and its conclusion runs contrary to the preponderance of scientific analysis.[20] Nevertheless, FWS used it to avoid listing trumpeter swans as endangered, and their population continues to dwindle as they fall victim to the tundra swan hunt.

To support its ruling, the agency also cited a 1987 peer-reviewed study of the tristate swan population. However, that study's principal author says that the agency seriously misinterpreted her findings.[21] Ruth Gale Shea, a wildlife biologist and expert on Rocky Mountain trumpeter swans, explains that her research led her to a conclusion opposite to that in the FWS determination; she found that the tristate population of trumpeter swans was notable for its reproductive isolation. "To date," Shea notes, "there are no data indicating that pairing with Canadian trumpeters is likely or that Canadian trumpeters will abandon their natal areas and fill in vacant tri-state breeding habitat as the tri-state population declines." Nonetheless, Shea says, the FWS selectively used only parts of her study to argue the precise opposite in support of the agency's ruling that the tristate trumpeters are not a discrete population segment.[22]

Following the January 2003 denial of protection to the tristate trumpeter swans, the nonprofit organization Public Employees for Environmental Responsibility (PEER) filed a complaint under the Data Quality Act of 2000. That act requires each federal agency to ensure and maximize "the quality, objectivity and integrity of information" it disseminates to the public and uses in its decision making.

PEER asked Williams to review the agency's ruling and its use of scientific information in the listing determination. PEER's request and subsequent appeal were both denied.[23] It turns out that Williams did convene a scientific panel to review the matter, and the panel's assessment, made available only after PEER filed a Freedom of Information Act request, unanimously recommended that the director grant the appeal, concurring with PEER that the agency's policy should not have been based upon a non-peer-reviewed document: "This panel concludes that the Dubovsky-Cornely paper lacks the objectivity demanded [by the Data Quality Act] because it was not subjected to any clearly documented quality assurance process, such as independent peer review."[24] In fact, in a letter to PEER, Williams agreed to ask the regional FWS office to obtain a peer review of the controversial Dubovsky-Cornely paper.[25]

Yet, despite authorizing the peer review, in March 2004 Williams overruled his own scientific panel's unanimous recommendation. He denied PEER's appeal and continued to refuse protection to the tristate trumpeter swan, despite overwhelming evidence that the agency's policy is based on inaccurate, misinterpreted, and questionable scientific information.[26]

PANTHER CHARADE

According to a Fish and Wildlife Service biologist who also serves on an FWS advisory panel, agency officials also knowingly used flawed science in assessing whether the Florida panther is endangered. The reason: to facilitate proposed economic development in southwestern florida.

Andrew Eller Jr., who has worked at the U.S. Fish and Wildlife Service for seventeen years, charges that his superiors knowingly inflated data about panther population viability and minimized assessments of the species' habitat needs.[27] Frustrated in his efforts to get FWS to correct its scientifically inaccurate assessments, he filed a legal complaint against the government under the Data Quality Act of 2000.[28] Eller, who worked for the past decade in Florida's Panther Recovery Program, said he filed the complaint because he "could no longer tolerate the scientific charade in which U.S. Fish and Wildlife Service officials are trying to pretend that the Florida panther is not in jeopardy."[29]

Eller charges that FWS assessments have inflated estimates of Florida panther populations by erroneously assuming that all known panthers are breeding adults, discounting the presence of juvenile, aged, and ill animals. In addition, he charges, FWS has knowingly minimized assessments of the Florida panthers' habitat needs by equating daytime habitat use patterns (when the panther is at rest) with nighttime habitat use patterns (when the panther is most active).[30]

Jane Comiskey, a University of Tennessee biologist and one of ten outside experts empanelled by FWS to help develop a conservation strategy for the panther, concurs with Eller. She adds that FWS has been unwilling to correct its misinformation despite repeated appeals by her panel.

Eller and Comiskey contend that the members of the FWS scientific review panel on the matter documented these and other serious errors in the agency's Conservation Strategy study of the Florida panther and unanimously urged that errors be corrected.[31] This peer-reviewed analysis was provided to the agency in November 2002 and February 2003. The U.S. Fish and Wildlife Service's response was to take the review panel's report off its website and to remove the agency's name from the analysis that the review panel filed in conjunction with Florida's Fish and Wildlife Conservation Commission.[32]

Meanwhile, Eller asserts, FWS has knowingly continued to disseminate the inaccurate information. As his complaint puts it: "The U.S. Fish and Wildlife Service's policy contends that no development project in southwest Florida constitutes jeopardy for the panther; the agency is simply relying on science that they know has been discredited."[33]

Comiskey adds that, as an independent scientific adviser, she hasn't been allowed to do the job the federal government hired her to do. As she notes, "It is hard to understand how an agency charged with using the best available science to protect panthers could object to correcting known errors. . . . There are certainly legitimate interests that may conflict with those of Florida's panthers, but those conflicts should be resolved through public policy channels, not by knowingly distorting panther science."[34]

Eller won his challenge under the Data Quality Act, but it remains to be seen if the agency will alter its policies to protect endangered panthers in Florida. Meanwhile, in retaliation for speaking out, FWS fired Eller in November 2004, the day after Bush's reelection. In an out-of-court settlement, he managed to get reinstated as an employee of the U.S. Fish and Wildlife Service, although, at his request, he will move to a new position.

MEET CRAIG MANSON

As we have seen, a favored Bush administration tactic is to put loyal "enforcers" in key midlevel positions—well placed to control scientific work on particular topics or at a given agency. Philip Cooney played such a role in censoring government research on global warming. Jeffrey Holmstead stifled and distorted scientific research on air pollution. Stephen Griles undermined the environmental assessment process to aid his former colleagues in the coal industry. When it comes to endangered species, a key Bush operative is Craig Manson, assistant secretary for Fish and Wildlife and Parks. Manson has been repeatedly accused of suppressing or manipulating scientific studies.[35]

Manson's heavy-handed approach extends beyond disputes over individual endangered species. Take the long-standing fight over the management of the nation's longest waterway, the Missouri River. On the one hand, farmers and barge owners want the river's flow to be uniform in the spring, summer, and fall so they can navigate the river and get grain to market. On the other hand, conservationists and others concerned about the health of the river's ecosystem favor a more natural management scheme in which the water fluctuates with the seasons, thereby aiding the spawning of fish and nesting of birds.

In late 2000, a group of biologists that had been studying the river flow on behalf of the U.S. Fish and Wildlife Service issued its "final biological opinion" on the matter, which was to take effect in 2003. This team had already issued preliminary findings that favored seasonal fluctuations in river flow, based on more than ten years of scientific research. Such a river management system, they contended, would comply with the Endangered Species Act by helping to protect two species of birds (the threatened piping plover and the endangered interior least tern) and one species of fish (the endangered pallid sturgeon). The team's findings had been confirmed by independent peer review as well as by the National Academy of Sciences.[36]

At this point, Craig Manson intervened on behalf of the Bush administration to stop the proposed environmental measures.[37] Unhappy with the results of the first team, Manson created a new review team, which revised the earlier biological opinion. In a memo, he described this new group as a "SWAT team" intended to review the situation and reach a swift judgment on the matter.[38]

After significant criticism from the press, environmental groups, and upper Missouri River basin elected officials, Assistant Secretary Manson added two scientists from the original team to his fifteen-member team, but neither of the new team's co-leaders had experience with the Missouri River or its issues.[39] In December 2003, the "SWAT team" released its amendment to the 2003 biological opinion, without peer review by independent experts.[40]

The amended opinion concluded that current Missouri flows did not threaten piping plovers or least terns, but it agreed that the proposed water levels for 2004 would jeopardize the pallid sturgeon. The amendment's proposed "reasonable and prudent alternatives" were significantly less stringent than the original biological opinion but did require the Army Corps of Engineers (the federal agency that manages water flows on the Missouri River) to modify river flow somewhat.[41]

Taking into account the amended biological opinion from the Fish and Wildlife Service, the Army Corps then developed an environmental impact statement and a new Master Manual (the plan that guides river management), which it released in March 2004. The Corps' plan does not restore the more natural ebb and flow of the river to protect threatened and endangered birds and fish, as recommended by the scientists on the original, peer-reviewed biological opinion; instead, it creates a plan to build new habitat for endangered pallid sturgeon.[42]

Absent independent peer review for the amended biological opinion, it is difficult to ascertain whether this opinion and plan will effectively protect the species at risk. What is clear is that a political agenda interfered once again with the scientific integrity of the policymaking process.

Allyn Sapa, a biologist who recently retired from the U.S. Fish and Wildlife Service, commented about this whole affair, "It's hard not to think that because our findings don't match up with what they want to hear, they are putting a new team on the job who will give them what they want."[43] Sapa had supervised the Missouri River project for more than five years.

Not surprisingly, Manson makes no secret of the fact that endangered species don't concern him much, despite his governmental position as one of their top protectors. As he said at a public conference: "If we are saying that the loss of species in and of itself is inherently bad, I don't think we know enough about how the world works to say that." In an interview, he explained that the extinction of species can be seen merely as artificial circumstances that are aiding a process of Darwinian natural selection. "The orthodoxy is that every species has a place in the ecosystem and therefore the loss of any species diminishes us in some negative way," Manson noted. "That's the orthodoxy. . . . But it's a presumptuous thing to suggest that we know for sure that that is a fact."[44]

FISH TALE

Similar tactics to undermine the Endangered Species Act extend beyond the confines of the U.S. Fish and Wildlife Service. Consider the case of six leading marine scientists asked by the National Marine Fisheries Service of the National Oceanic and Atmospheric Administration (NOAA) to review the status of endangered salmon stocks. These researchers found their science-based recommendations stripped from their official report.[45] As Robert Paine, the world-renowned ecologist who served as the panel's lead scientist, explains, "We were told to either strip out our recommendations or see our report end up in a drawer."[46]

Further, Paine and his panel contend that the new policy on endangered fish stocks put forth by NOAA, which is a division of the U.S. Department of Commerce, distorts the scientific evidence regarding the role of hatchery fish in maintaining viable populations of salmon in the Northwest.[47] The new policy refers to old or discredited information in contradiction to more up-to-date scientific information provided by the science advisory panel.

The controversy began in 2001, with a federal district court ruling about listing coastal coho salmon in Oregon under the Endangered Species Act. Before this ruling, the National Marine Fisheries Service (NMFS) had determined protection policies based on the numbers of wild salmon and steelhead populations, excluding hatchery-bred fish.[48] However, in a controversial verdict, the court ruled that the government's tallies should include hatchery-bred fish, despite evolutionarily significant differences.

Paine's group, the Salmon Recovery Science Review Panel, with membership approved by the National Research Council, was then asked by NOAA to study the situation. Providing extensive scientific documentation, this panel found a scientific basis for distinguishing between wild salmon and hatchery-raised fish of similar genetic stock. NMFS deleted this central recommendation from its final report on the grounds that it was policy, not science.

But according to panel member Ransom Myers, a marine biologist at Dalhousie University, "a massive amount of research shows that domestication occurs rapidly in hatchery fish." As Myers explains, "Within a few generations, these fish quickly evolve into something different, and lose their ability to survive in the wild."[49]

In NOAA's own words, the review panel was convened "to guide the scientific and technical aspects of recovery planning for listed salmon and steelhead species throughout the West Coast." In particular, the panel was instructed to "ensure that well accepted and consistent ecological and evolutionary principles form the basis for all [salmon and steelhead trout] recovery efforts."[50]

However, the agency apparently had other ideas in mind. The protected status of wild salmon and steelhead populations has been challenged by developers, farmers, ranchers, timber interests, and private property advocates, who seek to end government restrictions on land and water use to protect wild fish habitat. At the same time, the development of a new Bush administration policy on hatchery fish was being overseen by Mark Rutzick, whom President Bush appointed early in 2003 as special adviser to the NOAA general counsel.[51] Previously, Rutzick had served as a lawyer for the timber industry, and he was a strong opponent of the fish and wildlife protections that logging companies viewed as overly restrictive. Rutzick first proposed the strategy of including hatchery fish in population counts for endangered salmon while he worked on behalf of timber interests.[52]

Rutzick's apparent conflict of interest came to light amid a great deal of media attention in April and May 2005.[53] A copy of the draft policy leaked to the *Washington Post* suggested that all twenty-six listed populations of Northwest salmon and steelhead trout would be susceptible to de-listing under the Endangered Species Act once hatchery fish were included in their population assessments. The negative media coverage and public outcry subsequently led the NOAA administrator, Conrad Laut-enbacher, to assure senators and representatives from the Northwest that the new hatchery fish policy would not lead to de-listing and that his agency would maintain protections for at least twenty-five of the twenty-six listed populations.[54]

On May 28, 2005, the National Marine Fisheries Service released its proposed hatchery policy for publication in the *Federal Register*.[55] The new policy fails to include measurable scientific criteria for distinguishing hatchery fish from wild fish and, therefore, considers hatchery fish as part of natural populations. According to Jim Lichatowich, a salmon expert and former NMFS scientist, the new policy is "setting salmon recovery back about one hundred years."[56] While there appears to be a great deal of scientific documentation in the new policy and a number of supporting documents are included with the proposals, most of the science is old, and much of it was discredited or updated by the extensive efforts of the Salmon Recovery Science Review Panel's report, which is not included in the documentation.

In applying the new policy, NOAA has simultaneously issued for public comment a proposal for redefining and relisting twenty-seven varieties of salmon and steelhead in the Northwest.[57] Thus, while the new policy does not call for de-listing, it provides little protection against legal challenges to de-list populations that are threatened or endangered.

Lichatowich compares the inclusion of hatchery and wild fish in the same so-called Evolutionarily Significant Unit (as the Bush administration's proposed policy does) to lumping humans and chimpanzees into a similar grouping: "Like humans and chimps, hatchery fish have quite similar genetic make-up to their wild cousins, but to call them the same animal is scientifically inaccurate."[58]

The suppression of the advisory panel's recommendations led its members to publish their findings independently in the journal *Science*.[59] Describing the six scientists as "top-notch," the editor of *Science*, Donald Kennedy, noted that the article easily withstood review by scientific peers before publication. "Differences on scientific issues should be argued on the merits," Kennedy said about this incident, "and censorship isn't the way to conduct an honest debate."[60]

7

Burying More Than Intelligence

> The Bush administration has declared war on science. . . . In George
> Bush's America, ignorance is strength.
>
> HOWARD DEAN, "Bush's War on Science," *Daily Camera,* July 5, 2004

National security presents special issues for the federal government's
handling of scientific and technical information, as well as basic intelligence gathering. Without reliable factual data and impartial
analysis, government officials are in danger of misidentifying and mis-
interpreting threats to the nation. As a result, they risk building costly
weapons systems of little utility or deploying troops under false or mistaken pretexts. Perhaps the most serious misuse of intelligence by the
Bush administration lies outside strict matters of science, but because the
buildup to the war in Iraq can be seen as both a consequence and an example of the same mentality that has suppressed and undermined government science, I include it in my review. Even a cursory review of the
Bush administration's handling of technical information and analysis in
the national security realm raises a host of troubling questions.

Consider, for instance, the Bush administration's actions at the Department of Energy's National Nuclear Security Administration (NNSA),
the federal agency responsible for maintaining the nation's nuclear
weapons stockpile and overseeing the design and safety of the U.S. nuclear
arsenal. When Congress established the NNSA as a semi-autonomous en-
tity within the Department of Energy in 2000, it also created an independent technical advisory committee. This committee, formed in 2001,
had a membership of fifteen of the nation's most distinguished physicists

and technical experts with extensive knowledge of nuclear weapons, as well as former government officials and retired senior military officers.[1] In June 2003, the Bush administration summarily abolished the advisory committee.[2]

The abrupt termination of the committee startled many in the security establishment because virtually every administration from the dawn of the nuclear age has understood that the technically complex and highly secret mission of safeguarding and upholding the U.S. nuclear deterrent requires the advice of outstanding experts independent of the government. With each member handpicked by the NNSA administrator, the committee was created to "provide advice and recommendations on matters of technology, policy, and operation." The charter also indicated that the advisory group "is expected to be needed on a continuing basis."[3]

As Representative Edward Markey (D-MA) put it, the Bush administration had "disbanded the [government's] one forum for honest, unbiased external review of its nuclear weapons policies."[4] But Linton Brooks, the Bush administration's NNSA administrator, defended the abolition of the committee. The administration had "no shortage of advice," Brooks said, adding that "there are a lot of physicists who work" at the nation's weapons labs.[5]

The significance of this move by the Bush administration became clearer in 2004, when it was revealed that a report by the expert panel, finalized in March 2002, was being suppressed by the Bush administration despite the fact that the panel's reports were required by law to be public and unclassified.[6] A year after the panel had been disbanded and more than two years after the report was written, its recommendations were finally released under a Freedom of Information Act request, submitted by *Global Security Newswire*, which is sponsored by a nonprofit group called Nuclear Threat Initiative.

The advisory committee report was, among other things, critical of the Bush administration's plans to build so-called bunker buster nuclear weapons, a proposed new class of low-yield earth-penetrating nuclear weapons intended to target and destroy deeply buried and hardened facilities. The panel's experts noted that while the Bush administration's plans for this new variety of nuclear weapon "did not involve any radical departures from previously considered (or even implemented) systems" or offer new military capabilities, the program was enormously expensive, costing, by their estimate, as much as $485 million to develop. Committee members also complained that "concepts that have been discussed quite forcefully in recent times have yet to be examined in sufficient technical depth to determine that their potential military benefits justify the costs involved." Before moving forward, the panel recommended that "any new design concept should be thoroughly vetted by a critical and independent review that takes into account technical and other (e.g., military, training, etc.) considerations."[7] Nonetheless, President Bush's budget for fiscal year 2004 included $15 million for research on the Robust Nuclear Earth Penetrator (RNEP)—the nuclear bunker busters.

In addition to their critique in the report, some of the physicists on the committee had published articles on the bunker buster weapon system issue, explaining that nuclear weapons have only a limited capability to destroy deeply buried targets and, furthermore, that such attacks would inevitably produce a great deal of radioactive fallout. This is not a controversial opinion; experts at the national nuclear weapons laboratories agree that these effects are a relatively simple and well-understood consequence of basic physics.[8] Nevertheless, the panelists reported that a senior NNSA official expressed displeasure about the articles to the authors, presumably because the Bush administration's 2001 Nuclear Posture Review had called for the development of such weapons.

Government secrecy on security matters makes it hard to uncover all the particulars of this case. But, following an all-too-familiar pattern, it seems clear that when the Bush administration encountered expert analysis that dissented from its predetermined policy goals, it suppressed that analysis and ultimately removed the dissenters from the government altogether.

The NNSA incident is telling, but the fact is, the Bush administration began to spurn independent scientific and technical advice on security matters almost from the start. In 2001, for example, Bush administration officials dismissed the scientific committee that advised the State Department on technical matters related to arms control. The committee had been chaired by the physicist Richard Garwin, who had served on the Presidential Scientific Advisory Committee and the Defense Science Board under administrations of both parties and has for decades been a consultant to the national nuclear weapons laboratories and intelligence agencies. After this committee was dismissed, John R. Bolton, then undersecretary of state for arms control and international security, told Garwin that a new committee would be formed. But no such committee was ever appointed.[9] And it was about this time, in April 2001, that President Bush announced the United States intended to abandon the 1972 Antiballistic Missile Treaty so it could move quickly to develop a massive and long-contested ballistic missile defense system.

FAITH-BASED MISSILE DEFENSE

Once he had abrogated the Antiballistic Missile Treaty, President Bush ordered the deployment of a new missile defense system by the fall of 2004, even though most independent experts claimed that a reliable system could not be made operational within that three-year time frame.[10] And indeed, the record shows that Bush administration officials suppressed scientific evidence on the feasibility of the missile defense program and have ultimately deployed the costly and unproven system despite its repeated failures in Pentagon tests.

To accomplish this, the Bush administration ignored advice from experts inside and outside the military, as well as the dismal performance data yielded by Pentagon tests about the missile defense system's components. In 2002, for instance, Paul Wolfowitz, then deputy secretary of defense, told the Senate Appropriations Committee that prototype interceptors would be deployed by September 2004 and that they would be able to shoot down enemy missiles.[11] In Senate testimony in March 2003, Edward Aldridge, the Bush administration's undersecretary of defense, elaborated on the administration's plan. Like Wolfowitz, Aldridge was doubtless sending a signal from the Bush administration to the North Koreans, who were believed at the time to possess not only nuclear weapons but also intercontinental ballistic missiles with the potential to hit Alaska or possibly even the continental United States. Aldridge told the Senate panel that, by the end of 2004, the system would be "90 percent effective" in intercepting missiles from the Korean peninsula.[12]

This statement, however, was 100 percent implausible. No less an authority than Philip Coyle, who served as the Pentagon's top weapons tester during the 1990s, had reported in July 2001 that an effective missile defense system was "at least a decade" from completion.[13] In addition, in April 2003, shortly after Aldridge's Senate testimony, a report by the Government Accountability Office (GAO) found the Bush administration's missile defense plan unworkable and even dangerous. According to the report, the "performance of the system remains uncertain and unverified."[14]

Despite the assertions of the Bush administration, the U.S. missile defense system has not had a successful test since October 2002, and even that one was of dubious merit. In that test, a prototype interceptor was launched from the Ronald Reagan Missile Site in the Marshall Islands. Some 140 miles above the Pacific, the interceptor collided with a dummy warhead fired from the central California coast. The feat certainly sounded impressive. But, as Coyle noted, the test was "more scripted than a modern political convention." Not only did the Pentagon teams know the precise time of the staged attack, a transponder on the target missile emitted signals that ground control used to aim the interceptor.[15]

That was the "successful" test. In the last two trials, in December 2004 and February 2005, when engineers tried to use the same technology, *which the military has since deployed in Alaska,* the interceptors failed to even get off the ground.[16]

Of course, none of these testing results takes into account one of the strongest arguments critics have made about the infeasibility of missile defense: that the use of simple decoys by an enemy could easily foil even a fully functional system.[17] This argument, among others, has consistently led top analysts to doubt the utility of a missile defense system. As the editors of *Scientific American* stated succinctly in 2001: "Regarding missile defense, researchers' best guess is that a reliable system is infeasible."[18]

The Bush administration's strategy in the face of such obstacles? It ignored the critiques of technical experts and ordered the Pentagon to field the missile defense system without even establishing detailed performance standards, not to mention meeting them.[19]

According to one report, by the end of 2005, the Bush administration planned to have sixteen antimissile launchers deployed at Fort Greely, Alaska, and another four at Vandenberg Air Force Base on the central California coast.[20] As of April 2006, roughly half of these interceptors

are in place. In the event of an attack, the unproven system must identify, track, and intercept a warhead as small as five feet long traveling
some 15,000 miles per hour. The operators of the system in Alaska will
have somewhere between three and five minutes after an enemy missile
is launched to accomplish the task.[21]

Of course, the goal of missile defense long predates the Bush administration.[22] The U.S. government has actively pursued it as a research
program since it was first proposed by former president Ronald Reagan.
No administration, however, has embraced the program as has the Bush
administration or tried to bring it to the battlefield by sheer force of will.
Already, the Bush administration has spent some $25 billion on the mis-
sile defense program, and it plans to spend an additional $55 billion by
2011. The spending has now ramped up to around $10 billion annually,
more than twice as much as is being spent on any other weapons system.[23]

Despite this enormous outlay, there is no indication that the missile
defense system will have any military utility whatsoever, even with
major modifications in the field. "The system . . . has no demonstrated
capability to defend the United States under realistic operational condi-
tions," Coyle says, adding that some twenty to thirty developmental hurdles remain before it could even be ready for realistic testing. Sur-
mounting each of these hurdles, he says, could take two to three years of
work apiece.[24] What kind of additional difficulties might ensue to put
these developmental components together in a cohesive system is anyone's guess. As the latest oversight report from the Government Accountability Office politely complained, time pressures from the Bush
administration to deploy the experimental and untested system caused
the Pentagon's Missile Defense Agency "to stray from a knowledge-
based acquisition strategy."[25]

Like the GAO, Coyle maintains that political considerations, and not
technical merit, are driving the Bush administration's program.[26] Sadly,
though, the detailed critique Coyle compiled during his tenure as the
Pentagon's director of Operational Test and Evaluation has been classified retroactively by the Bush administration, despite protests by members of the House Committee on Government Reform.[27]

Thomas Christie, Coyle's successor at the Pentagon's testing and evaluation office, has also expressed concern about the Bush administration's

missile defense program. Christie's annual report for fiscal year 2004 states that the components of the missile defense system "remain immature," making it impossible to "estimate the current mission capability of the BMDS [Ballistic Missile Defense System] with high confidence." Any such assessment, the report complains, will thus necessarily have to "rely heavily on models and simulations of individual elements." In addition, the report notes, "The lack of flight-testing has delayed the validation and accreditation of some key performance models and simulations."[28] Even Christie's relatively mild criticisms have been squelched, however. The Bush administration has quietly removed the past three years' worth of annual reviews by Christie from the Pentagon's website.[29]

The Bush administration persistently mandates—presumably through Defense Secretary Donald Rumsfeld—that the Pentagon present a rosy picture. Testifying before Congress in the spring of 2005, Gen. James Cartwright, commander of the U.S. Strategic Command, said: "In an emergency, we are, in fact, in the position that we are confident that we can operate the system."[30]

When a reporter from the *Seattle Times* questioned Lt. Col. Gregory Bowen, the commander of the 49th Missile Defense Battalion at Fort Greely, Alaska, where the system has been fielded, however, the story was strikingly different. "Does the capability exist this minute to shoot if we see something? The answer to that is no," Bowen said. "So when the generals are saying, 'Yes, we could shoot this thing now,' what they mean is, if the system is put on alert we can shoot now," said Bowen, adding with a wry smile: "And if I contradict anything the generals have said, they're right."[31] Meanwhile, the Pentagon will not say how long it would take to place the system on alert, and Defense Secretary Rumsfeld has postponed indefinitely the decision of when to authorize the alert status.[32]

STOVEPIPING IRAQ INTELLIGENCE

The Bush administration has spent tens of billions of U.S. taxpayer dollars to deploy an utterly unproven and dubious missile defense system, but this pales in comparison to the cost of the war in Iraq. The Iraq war—and the mishandling of technical information and intelligence that led to it—will undoubtedly go down in history as the most egregious of the Bush administration's failings. The picture will surely become clearer in time as more of the administration's now-classified deliberations are made public, but already an astonishingly strong and disturbing case has emerged in the significant number of governmental and journalistic accounts that have appeared to date.

Strictly speaking, intelligence gathering is distinct from the government's handling of other kinds information and ought to be seen as a special case. The field is greatly complicated by the ever-present issues of secrecy and uncertainty that attend all intelligence work. Analysts always face the difficult task of weighing the accuracy of intelligence information deriving from varied and often suspect sources. Nonetheless, it is essential to review here at least a few of the particulars of the lead-up to the Iraq war because they so closely fit the Bush administration's disturbing pattern in which ideology triumphs over data and factual analysis. Much of this intelligence work, after all, involves the government's handling of the most sensitive kinds of scientific and technical information, from the analysis of satellite reconnaissance data to the verification of official documents.

The Bush administration's gross mishandling of intelligence information leading to the Iraq war can be seen to mirror the apparent disdain for facts the administration has exhibited in so many other fields. In this case, however, the consequences have been even more costly, leading to tens of thousands of deaths, the dramatic decline of the stature of the United States in the eyes of the world community, and the expenditure of roughly a billion dollars in U.S. taxpayer dollars *every week* the Iraq occupation continues.[33]

To understand this story, it is important to recognize, first of all, that the Bush administration decided to invade Iraq long before it made its decision known to Congress or the American public. This is now clear from many sources. In Ron Suskind's book *The Price of Loyalty,* for instance, former Treasury secretary Paul O'Neill describes the first major national security meeting of the Bush administration on January 30, 2001—nearly nine months before the terrorist attacks of September 11. O'Neill recounts that, at that meeting, Bush tasked Secretary of Defense Donald Rumsfeld and Chairman of the Joint Chiefs of Staff General H. Hugh Shelton with examining military options in Iraq, including rebuilding the military coalition from the 1991 Gulf War, and exploring "how it might look" to use U.S. ground forces in the north and the south of Iraq. In Suskind's words, "Ten days in, and it was about Iraq."[34]

The terrorist attacks of September 11, 2001, gave the administration's fixation on Iraq added urgency as well as political cover. Richard Clarke, the Bush administration's senior counterterrorism expert on the National Security Council who served in four separate administrations, recounted Bush's concerted effort to link Saddam Hussein to the attacks. In his book *Against All Enemies: Inside America's War on Terror,* Clarke recounts that, on the evening of September 12, 2001, Bush "grabbed a few of us and closed the door to the conference room. 'Look,' he told us, 'I know you have a lot to do and all . . . but I want you, as soon as you can, to go back over everything, everything. See if Saddam did this. See if he's linked in any way.'" When Clarke protested that it was clearly an Al Qaeda operation, Bush insisted, "Just look. I want to know any shred . . . Look into Iraq, Saddam."[35]

Perhaps most damning, though, is the notorious Downing Street Memo. This secret British document, leaked to the press in 2005, reports on a July 2002 meeting of key British cabinet and other officials, held when Sir Richard Dearlove, head of the British intelligence service, MI6, returned from a trip to Washington. It reveals that the Bush administration had, at that point, already made the decision to go to war. "Military action was now seen as inevitable," the memo states. According to Dearlove: "Bush wanted to remove Saddam, through military action, justified by the conjunction of terrorism and WMD [weapons of mass destruction]. *But the intelligence and facts were being fixed around the policy*" (emphasis added).[36]

A picture emerges from numerous insider accounts of how this "fixing" of intelligence occurred within the Bush administration. The story begins with a small, tight-knit group of zealous neoconservatives for whom the goal of toppling Iraq's Saddam Hussein was paramount. The group included Vice President Dick Cheney, Undersecretary of Defense for Policy Douglas Feith, Undersecretary of State for Arms Control John Bolton, and Deputy Secretary of Defense Paul Wolfowitz. Also intimately involved were Secretary of Defense Donald Rumsfeld, CIA director George Tenet, National Security Adviser Condoleezza Rice, and a number of other well-positioned administration officials.[37]

As we now know, several members of this group—especially Feith and Bolton—disdained and mistrusted much of the work of the U.S. intelligence community, especially on Iraq. As a result, they bypassed normal intelligence procedures to amass a case for the invasion of Iraq that fit the administration's predetermined policy. For instance, Greg Thielmann, an intelligence expert with the State Department's Bureau of Intelligence and Research, recalls that, a few months after George W. Bush took office, he was appointed as the daily intelligence liaison to John Bolton. As Seymour Hersh recounts in a detailed article in the *New Yorker*, Thielmann says he soon found himself shut out of Bolton's staff meetings. "I was intercepted at the door of his office and told, 'the undersecretary doesn't need you to attend this meeting anymore.' " When Thielmann protested that he was there to provide intelligence input, the aide reportedly said, "The undersecretary wants to keep this in the family."[38]

Karen Kwiatkowski, a lieutenant colonel in the U.S. Air Force who retired in July 2003 after twenty years of service in the military, also offers a particularly blunt inside assessment of the way prewar intelligence about Iraq was "fixed" to conform to the administration's decision to invade Iraq. At the end of her tour of duty, Kwiatkowski served under Douglas Feith in the Near East and South Asia (NESA) directorate of the Pentagon's policy arm. During this period, from May 2002 until February 2003, the Bush administration established the Pentagon's so-called Office of Special Plans (OSP), which conducted its own prewar intelligence gathering. As Kwiatkowski reports, "I observed firsthand the formation of the Pentagon's Office of Special Plans and watched the latter stages of the neoconservative capture of the policy-intelligence nexus in the run-up to the invasion of Iraq. This seizure of the reins of U.S. Middle East policy was directly visible to many of us working the Near East and South Asia policy office, and yet there seemed to be little any of us could do about it."[39]

During the period Kwiatkowski was stationed there, she says, OSP kept expanding under the purview of Douglas Feith, a man who, she and many others claim, had a dramatically partisan approach to intelligence gathering. Disdaining the normal work of the U.S. intelligence community as overly cautious, Feith established his own ad hoc intelligence-gathering effort clearly aimed at building a case for war. According to

Kwiatkowski, Feith sought only information, however questionable, that bolstered the case for an Iraq invasion. It has also come to light that Feith caused the CIA to postpone its assessment of Iraq's link to terrorism after a personal visit to CIA headquarters at which he raised numerous objections to a draft CIA report. And while the CIA was revising its assessment, Feith's team went directly to the White House to give an "alternative briefing" to Vice President Dick Cheney's chief of staff and to National Security Adviser Condoleezza Rice's deputy in which Feith alleged there were "fundamental problems" with CIA intelligence gathering on Iraq's connection to Al Qaeda.[40]

Through such aggressive tactics, Feith, Bolton, and others established a climate that thwarted dissent about the administration's war plans. As Kwiatkowski recalls: "I was present at a staff meeting when Bill Luti [assistant secretary of defense for NESA who served under Feith] called Marine general and former chief of Central Command Anthony Zinni a 'traitor,' because Zinni had publicly expressed reservations about the rush to war." Operating as a renegade intelligence-gathering arm and shunning the expertise available within the intelligence community, the OSP called the shots. "War is generally crafted and pursued for political reasons, but the reasons given to the Congress and to the American people for this one were inaccurate and so misleading as to be false. Moreover," Kwiatkowski charges, "they were false by design."[41]

Kenneth Pollack, a National Security Council expert on Iraq during the Clinton administration, who presented a strong case for invading Iraq in his 2002 book *The Threatening Storm,* also criticized the Bush administration's intelligence operation regarding Iraq. As Pollack put it, the Bush administration "dismantle[d] the existing filtering process that for fifty years had been preventing the policymakers from getting bad information. They created 'stovepipes' to get the information they wanted directly to the top leadership."[42]

The result of this "stovepiping" was that officials at the highest levels of the Bush administration were able to "cherry pick" raw intelligence information—often from highly questionable sources—to support their predetermined policy of invasion. It also meant that top Bush officials—including the president and the vice president—regularly repeated largely unsubstantiated intelligence claims, including that a link existed between Saddam Hussein and Al Qaeda; that Iraq possessed mobile bioweapons laboratories and vast arsenals of chemical weapons; and, in one of the most notorious and disturbing claims, that Iraq had sought to purchase uranium from Niger in 1999 to build nuclear weapons.

"DEAD WRONG"

The twisted story of the Bush administration's false claims about Iraq's interest in Niger's uranium has been treated at length in many other sources, including the 500-page review by the U.S. Senate Select Committee on Intelligence in July 2004, as well as the Robb-Silbermann Presidential Commission on Intelligence Capabilities of the United States Regarding Weapons of Mass Destruction. According to the Senate committee, the Niger uranium story was one of the key points on which the Bush administration was "dead wrong" in its intelligence assessment about Iraq.[43] As of this writing, the case and its aftermath are also the subject of ongoing investigations by the FBI and a federal grand jury.[44]

While the entire story has yet to be disclosed, much has already come to light. We now know that this bogus piece of intelligence was based, at least in part, on forged documents that were originally passed by a retired member of Italian military intelligence named Rocco Martino to an Italian journalist who turned them over to the U.S. embassy in Rome in 2002.[45] The documents—some twenty-two photocopied pages—purported to corroborate Iraqi interest in purchasing uranium "yellowcake" from Niger in 1999.

We also know that the documents were easy for trained intelligence experts to identify as forgeries. On March 7, 2003, just days before the U.S.-led invasion of Iraq, when analysts at the International Atomic Energy Agency (IAEA) finally received the documents, they were reportedly able to determine within a matter of hours that they were fakes. Using little more than a Google search, IAEA experts discovered a host of obvious flaws. The documents used an obsolete letterhead from the Niger government and listed incorrect names of Niger officials. One document, purportedly from 1999, for example, bore the signature of Allele Elhadj Habibou, Niger's foreign minister from a decade earlier.[46]

There is a good deal of circumstantial evidence that many in the U.S. intelligence community may have also recognized the documents as forgeries—and in the context of this book, it is worth noting the technical nature of the methods used to determine their inauthenticity.[47] But, from the moment the forged Niger documents appeared, they were stovepiped and embraced by the pro-war faction within the Bush administration. And, in the intelligence climate the administration created, knowledge in the intelligence community that the information was suspect did not stop it from being publicly disclosed at the highest levels of the administration and even included in President Bush's January 2003 State of the Union address.

It is also known that, early in 2002, the CIA dispatched former U.S. ambassador Joseph Wilson to Niger to investigate the claims about Iraq's interest in the country's uranium. On February 22, 2002, Wilson reported to the CIA and the State Department that the information was "unequivocally wrong." There was, he found, no evidence that Iraq had sought the uranium from Niger in 1999. But Wilson's findings were either overlooked or ignored by senior officials who didn't want to hear anything that ran counter to their predetermined policy objective.

Outraged, Wilson went public with his findings with an op-ed piece in the *New York Times* on July 6, 2003 (shortly after the U.S. invasion of Iraq had begun), entitled "What I Didn't Find in Africa." Wilson stated: "Based on my experience with the administration in the months leading up to the war, I have little choice but to conclude that some of the intelligence related to Iraq's nuclear weapons program was twisted to exaggerate the Iraqi threat."[48] In apparent retaliation for Wilson's public charges—in an effort that many believe was out of Vice President Cheney's office—the identity of Wilson's wife, Valerie Plame, who had served as an undercover CIA agent, was leaked to journalists. As of this writing, the subsequent federal grand jury investigation into this retaliation is still under way, even though the story of Iraq's purported uranium purchases has long since unraveled.

In the immediate run-up to the Iraq invasion in March 2003, it fell to U.S. secretary of state Colin Powell to present the Bush administration's charges against Iraq before the United Nations Security Council. Given the IAEA's unequivocal public debunking of the Niger-uranium documents, it is to Powell's credit that he removed mention of it from his presentation. Nonetheless, virtually every one of the other cherry-picked intelligence points Powell did make—from the alleged existence of mobile biological weapons labs to the alleged purpose of aluminum tubes Iraq tried to procure—has since been shown to be utterly false. And, of course, after Saddam Hussein was toppled, no nuclear weapons program—or weapon of mass destruction of any kind—was found in Iraq.

The outcome completely vindicated the work of the U.N. weapons inspectors. "The IAEA has now conducted a total of 218 nuclear inspections at 141 sites, including 21 that have not been inspected before," Mohamed ElBaradei, IAEA's director general, had told the U.N. Security Council at the time of Powell's presentation in 2002. "At this stage, the following can be stated: One, there is no indication of resumed nuclear activities in those buildings that were identified through the use of satellite imagery as being reconstructed or newly erected since 1998, nor any indication of nuclear-related prohibited activities at any inspected sites. Second, there is no indication that Iraq has attempted to import uranium since 1990."[49]

To be sure, Powell's performance at the U.N. had grave consequences. He says that he worked in earnest for four days to try to corroborate the information the White House told him to present. In 2005, after leaving the Bush administration, Powell publicly expressed his profound anger and regret over his role in dispensing false information. "I'm very sore," he says. "I'm the one who made the television moment. I was mightily disappointed when the sourcing of it all became very suspect and everything started to fall apart."[50]

Lawrence Wilkerson, Powell's chief of staff from 2002 through 2005, is even more blunt in his assessment. He says the information in Powell's presentation initially came from a White House document that "was anything but an intelligence document." According to Wilkerson, the White House presented Powell with a cobbled-together list of questionable allegations that he likens to "a Chinese menu" from which the White House intended Powell to "pick and choose" in making a case for war against Iraq. "I wish I had not been involved in it," Wilkerson says of the process leading up to Powell's presentation. "I look back on it, and I still say it was the lowest point in my life."[51]

MISREPRESENTING EVIDENCE ON IRAQ'S ALUMINUM TUBES

In the story of the Bush administration's handling of prewar intelligence about Iraq, it is instructive to look closely at one particular technical aspect: the way key officials selectively interpreted information about Iraq's alleged attempt to purchase aluminum tubes. The case shows how the administration appears to have knowingly disregarded scientific analysis of intelligence data that challenged its case.[52]

In the weeks leading up to the war, senior administration officials bolstered their case that Saddam Hussein had nuclear ambitions by repeatedly stating Iraq had attempted to acquire more than a hundred thousand high-strength aluminum tubes for gas centrifuges to be used for enriching uranium. (Highly enriched uranium is one of the two materials that can be used to make nuclear weapons.) There is no question that Iraq ordered the tubes from a factory in southern China. Rather, the question before the intelligence community was whether these tubes—which in fact never reached Iraq because of a successful U.S. interception—were meant to be used for centrifuges or as motor casings for short-range rockets.

Nonetheless, the claim that the tubes were for centrifuges was made unequivocally by National Security Adviser Condoleezza Rice, by Vice President Dick Cheney, and finally by President Bush, not only on September 12, 2002, in his address to the United Nations General Assembly, but on several other occasions, including his State of the Union address to Congress on January 28, 2003.[53]

The dominant insiders in the Bush administration, who had effectively commandeered control of the nation's intelligence-gathering operation, clearly favored the view that the tubes were intended for centrifuges. They put forward the argument that the tight tolerances on the tubes' dimensions and finish could have no other interpretation. However, some of the nation's most experienced intelligence officers and most technically capable analysts disagreed with this interpretation.

A set of technical experts from the Department of Energy's (DOE) Oak Ridge, Livermore, and Los Alamos National Laboratories reviewed the analysis of the tubes and determined that their dimensions were far from ideal for centrifuge use. A group within the State Department's Bureau of Intelligence and Research concurred. These experienced teams also noted that the dimensions and the aluminum alloy were identical to those of tubes Iraq had acquired for rockets in the 1980s.[54]

Furthermore, the Iraqis had developed and tested centrifuges before the first Gulf War that were much more capable than those that could have been built with the imported tubes. As one DOE analyst explained to Senate investigators, the tubes were so poorly suited for centrifuges that, if Iraq truly wanted to use them this way, it would be to our benefit to "just give them the tubes." The DOE experts also pointed out that if these tubes were actually intended for centrifuges, there should be evidence of attempts by the Iraqis to acquire hundreds of thousands of other very specific components that would also be needed, but no such evidence existed. This critique of the Bush administration's interpretation was seconded by the State Department's intelligence branch and, independently, by an international group of centrifuge experts advising the International Atomic Energy Agency.[55]

In fact, especially in retrospect, it is hard to see how the Bush administration could have managed to override these concerns and continue to contend that the tubes were evidence of Iraq's nuclear ambitions. The nation's top experts on the subject determined that the tubes were both too narrow and too thick for centrifuges. They were too shiny: they had been manufactured with an anodized coating that could react with uranium gas and make them wholly unsuitable for uranium enrichment. They were three times too long for use in a centrifuge unless Iraq wanted to follow a new and untested design. And finally, and perhaps most obviously, they were identical to tubes the Iraqis had previously purchased for use as rocket casings.

Despite all these objections made by U.S. intelligence officers, the Bush administration clung to the claim that the aluminum tubes were intended for the manufacture of uranium for nuclear weapons. And the claim was central to Secretary Powell's case before the United Nations that Iraq had a nuclear weapons program. He had been briefed by the IAEA about its disagreement with the Bush administration's analysis and was aware of a controversy inside the U.S. government about the administration's claim because the DOE and State Department had both commented on the draft of his speech. Yet Powell, on behalf of the Bush administration, dismissed this disagreement in his speech by lumping the U.S. experts with the Iraqis: "Other experts, and the Iraqis themselves, argue that they are really to produce the rocket bodies for a conventional weapon, a multiple rocket launcher," he said.[56] Many experts, especially at the Department of Energy, took Powell's wording as a particular slap in the face. "My friends in DOE felt shocked," one analyst said. "We were thrown in the same camp as the Iraqis."[57]

As Dr. David Albright, a weapons expert and president of the Institute for Science and International Security in Washington, DC, has noted, "This case serves to remind us that decision makers are not above misusing technical and scientific analysis to bolster their political goals. It bespeaks something seriously wrong that a proper technical adjudication of this matter was never conducted. There was certainly plenty of time to accomplish it."[58]

The willful misreading of intelligence information such as Iraq's real intended use for the aluminum tubes had grave consequences for the United States and the world. However, despite sharp critiques from the president's so-called 9/11 Commission and the Senate intelligence committee, the Bush administration has yet to issue any major reprimand or penalty to those responsible for the intelligence failures.

Quite the contrary.

Former CIA director George Tenet resigned, but President Bush subsequently awarded him the Medal of Freedom. Condoleezza Rice, who had primary responsibility as national security adviser to review the full extent of the government's intelligence on Iraq, has in the Bush administration's second term been elevated to secretary of state. John Bolton, who played a key role in intimidating intelligence analysts whose findings differed from what he wanted to hear and who participated in the stovepiping operation, has been promoted, in a controversial recess appointment, to a position as U.S. ambassador to the United Nations.

Equally telling are the consequences for two of the intelligence analysts at the heart of the fiasco—George Norris and Robert Campos of the army's National Ground Intelligence Center. Norris and Campos told the Bush administration what it wanted to hear. They did not seek or obtain information available from the nation's top experts at the Energy Department and elsewhere showing that the tubes were identical to a type used for years as rocket-motor cases by Iraq's military. Instead, they reported that the tubes were evidence of an Iraqi nuclear buildup. Their work was singled out by the Senate Intelligence committee for the "serious lapse in analytic tradecraft" it represented. And yet, in the strange world of the Bush administration, these analysts have been given performance awards—cash bonuses their department offers for excellence on the job—in each of the past three years.[59]

8

Stacking the Deck

> I don't think any administration has penetrated so deeply into the advisory committee structure as this one, and I think it matters. If you start picking people by their ideology instead of their scientific credentials, you are inevitably reducing the quality of the advisory group.
>
> DONALD KENNEDY, editor of *Science* and former president of Stanford University, January 2002

To some extent, the complaints raised about the Bush administration's lack of integrity on scientific and technical matters boil down to issues of fairness. Politicians often like to say the United States is a fair place because it is a nation of laws. But laws are only useful if there is a working system through which to enforce them. And as many critics have noted, the Bush administration has routinely circumvented laws it doesn't like by appointing to enforcement positions at federal agencies officials who have no intention of enforcing the law.

We have already reviewed the work of some of these "foxes in the henhouse," from Jeffrey Holmstead at the Environmental Protection Agency to Stephen Griles at the Department of the Interior. But the federal government is large; even the many anecdotes presented in this book barely scratch its surface. A number of interest groups have compiled lists of these kinds of Bush administration appointments. One report, published jointly by the Center for American Progress and OMB Watch, profiles nearly fifty Bush administration officials who have actively tried to undermine the previous work of the agencies to which they were appointed.

In addition to Holmstead and Griles, that list includes such Bush appointees as Samuel Bodman III, deputy secretary of commerce, who tried to stall governmental action on global warming in his position as chair of the federal Interagency Working Group on Climate Change Science and Technology; Rebecca Watson, assistant interior secretary for land and minerals management, who is now in charge of the enforcement of mining laws but who spent her entire legal career prior to the Bush administration representing the interests of the mining and timber industries; and Adam Sharp, who at the end of 2004 left his position overseeing government decisions about pesticides as EPA's associate assistant administrator for the Office of Prevention, Pesticides, and Toxics to return to lobbying for the American Farm Bureau Federation, which has consistently opposed environmental regulations on the agriculture industry.[1]

The appointment of so many strikingly partisan gatekeepers to mid-level federal positions represents a well-established and remarkably successful strategy by the Bush administration. But there is a related strategy with perhaps even more insidious results: the attempt to stack the nation's scientific advisory panels with people chosen for their political ideology rather than their professional expertise.

Previous chapters have touched on this issue. Chapter 3, for instance, discussed the Bush administration's handling of the Childhood Lead Poisoning Prevention Committee at the Centers for Disease Control. In that case, top Bush administration appointees at the Department of Health and Human Services (HHS) summarily dismissed or rejected some of the nation's leading experts on lead poisoning to empanel far less qualified candidates who had been recommended by lobbyists from the lead-paint industry. Chapter 4 reviewed the impact of the appointment of David Hager, the evangelical activist physician, to the Food and Drug Administration's Reproductive Health Advisory Committee. There Hager's religiously motivated intervention played a role in limiting American women's access to contraceptives.

To appreciate the impact of the politicization of the nation's science advisory committees, consider that nearly a thousand committees, panels, commissions, and councils advise the federal government on everything from how to allocate federal research dollars to what should be considered permissible levels of pesticide residue on produce.[2] Traditionally, appointments to these expert advisory groups have been relatively nonpartisan and merit based. Politics has always played some role in the selection process, but the federal government has largely avoided overt bias by relying predominantly on nominations by agency staff who, in conjunction with colleagues outside of government, tend to favor candidates widely recognized for their scientific expertise and reputation as leaders in their fields.

The balancing of scientific advisory positions in government is not only a matter of tradition but also one of law. According to the Federal Advisory Committee Act of 1972, the membership of federal advisory committees must be "fairly balanced in terms of the points of view represented and the functions to be performed by the advisory committee." In addition, the advisory process must "contain appropriate provisions to ensure that the advice and recommendations of the advisory committee will not be inappropriately influenced by the appointing authority or by any special interest, but will instead be the result of the advisory committee's independent judgment."[3]

The Bush administration has repeatedly asserted that it is upholding the spirit of balance. Responding to questions about irregularities in the appointment process early in 2003, for example, White House spokesperson Ken Lasaius stated that President Bush makes appointments "on the basis of putting the best qualified person into a position."[4] But the record shows that the current administration has repeatedly allowed political considerations to trump scientific qualifications in the appointment process.

Not only has the Bush administration picked candidates with questionable credentials for advisory positions, it has routinely used political litmus tests to vet candidates for even the least political of its government review panels. And it has regularly chosen candidates put forward by industry lobbyists over those recommended by its own federal agencies. This last charge is particularly troubling because industry executives are often also large campaign contributors. Such appointments leave the Bush administration open to charges of cronyism and corruption.

WHEN EVEN A NOBEL LAUREATE WON'T DO

Perhaps one of the most complete pictures of the Bush administration's politicization of the appointment process for scientific and technical advisers comes from a branch of the National Institutes of Health (NIH) called the Fogarty International Center. As its name suggests, the Fogarty Center develops international research and training programs to address global health issues, such as efforts to augment nutrition, vaccination, or AIDS prevention. Gerald T. Keusch, who served from October 1998 to December 2003 as director of the center as well as associate director for international research at the NIH, recounts a dramatic change in the appointment process when the Bush administration took office.

Keusch, who is now the assistant provost for global health at Boston University Medical Center, says that during his three years under the Bush administration, he proposed twenty-six candidates to serve on the Fogarty Center's advisory board. All the candidates he nominated were approved within a week by the NIH director. In almost every case, though, the Bush administration delayed each of Keusch's nominations for many months. In the end, administration officials only approved seven of them—rejecting the remaining nineteen candidates. By contrast, Keusch says, the Clinton administration swiftly approved all seven of the nominations he made during his tenure under that administration.

It bears noting that, despite whatever resentment Keusch may have felt about having so many of his nominees rejected, he went public with this information only after being sought out for questioning about the matter by the author of an article titled "Science, Politics, and Federal Advisory Committees" that appeared the *New England Journal of Medicine*.[5] Since that time, though, Keusch has provided further details about the matter that paint a troubling picture of the degree of politicization in the Bush administration's appointment process.

What is most notable about Keusch's disclosure is the impeccable credentials of the candidates he nominated. Because the Fogarty International Center gives research grants, Keusch says, "I knew what skills I needed on my board to review grants, and I knew who I thought would be the right people to do it."[6] For example, in his first set of nominations after Bush took office in 2001, Keusch proposed to empanel Thorsten Wiesel, a Nobel laureate in medicine; Jane Menken, a highly respected demographer at the University of Colorado; and Geeta Rao Gupta, an internationally known expert on women's health and the president of the Washington, DC–based International Center for Research on Women. After more than four months of delay in Secretary Tommy Thompson's office at HHS, Keusch said he learned that all three of these initial candidates had been rejected without explanation.

"I was extremely angry," Keusch recalls. He went to Yvonne Maddox, then acting deputy director of NIH, and demanded that the institute set up a meeting with Secretary Thompson's office.[7] As Keusch puts it, "I had managed to get a Nobel laureate to agree to serve on my board, and if he was going to be rejected, I wanted to know why."

When pressed for details about what followed, Keusch recounts that he found the meeting with Secretary Thompson's staff and other administration officials deeply disturbing. "There is no written record," Keusch says, "but I remember the meeting most clearly. I was told that Dr. Wiesel was rejected because he had signed too many full-page letters in the *New York Times* critical of President Bush. I was told Dr. Rao was unacceptable because she was on the board of the Alan Guttmacher Institute, the nonprofit reproductive health research organization. Dr. Menken, I was told, was deemed too political, although the only evidence I was given of this was that she was a registered Democrat."

Keusch reports that in one case even a sitting board member was rejected. When he sought to renew the term of Cutberto Garza, the associate provost at Cornell University and an expert on international nutrition, Secretary Thompson's office denied the request. Eventually, Keusch said, the experience was so frustrating that he stopped even talking to candidates in advance of their confirmation. "It was too embarrassing to me to get these top people to agree to serve as board members only to have to tell them they were rejected."

Keusch's testimony points to an unprecedented degree of politicization in the appointment process for people serving as scientific and technical advisers. He himself says that in his own experience, the difference between the administrations of George W. Bush and Bill Clinton "was like the difference between night and day."[8]

There is little question that, thanks to the partisan politics of the Bush administration, the nation was deprived of the technical expertise of Keusch's indisputably qualified nominees. One could make the case, of course, that an administration has the right to keep a close rein on appointments that might have significant policy ramifications. And it is true that the Fogarty Center's advisory board members arguably deal more directly with policy matters than some scientific advisory panels do. Unfortunately, however, the Bush administration has politicized even appointments that have virtually no bearing on policy matters.

According to the Government Accountability Office, roughly ten thousand people serve on the nation's scientific and technical advisory panels. A far greater number, though—as many as forty thousand—participate on boards that review the vast grant-making effort by the federal government that helps underwrite the nation's scientific research at universities and research institutions across the country. Examples of politicization have surfaced in this traditionally apolitical arena as well.

POLITICAL LITMUS TESTS ON WORKPLACE SAFETY PANEL

In one well-documented case, mentioned in chapter 1, Tommy Thompson, as secretary of Health and Human Services, dismissed three well-qualified experts on ergonomics from a narrowly focused peer review panel at the National Institute for Occupational Safety and Health (NIOSH). The three nominees in question had been selected to join a study section of the Advisory Committee on Occupational Safety and Health that evaluates research grants on workplace injuries.[9] Based on their credentials and reputations in the field, the three had been chosen by the committee chair and panel staff, and had initially been approved by the director of NIOSH. Study sections such as this one are responsible for offering peer review of ongoing research, not for advising on policy matters, and therefore have almost never seen their service affected by a change of administration. Traditionally, scientists in such positions have always been chosen strictly for their expertise, just as their peer review work requires them to assess research solely based on its scientific merit.

In this case, however, at least two of the rejected nominees believe that the Bush administration denied them positions because of their support for a workplace ergonomics standard, a policy opposed by the administration. Laura Punnett, a professor at the University of Massachusetts at Lowell, states she has little doubt that she was removed from the study section for political reasons. There were no complaints about her work during the year she served in an ad hoc basis on the study section, and she was told upon her dismissal by the chair of the study section that her removal had nothing to do with her credentials or the quality of her work.[10] "I was shocked," Punnett told the press after her rejection. "I think it conveys very powerfully that part of the goal is to intimidate researchers and limit what research questions are asked."[11]

Another rejected nominee, Manuel Gomez, the former director of scientific affairs at the American Industrial Hygiene Association, says he was not informed why his nomination was rejected after having been endorsed by NIOSH staff. He adds, however, that an agency staffer did tell him he "had never before seen this kind of decision coming in contravention of the agency's recommendation."[12]

Here again, the circumstances of the case strongly indicate a politically motivated intervention. Such concerns are heightened by the fact that another prospective member of the study section—Pamela Kidd, associate dean of the College of Nursing at Arizona State University—charged publicly that someone from Secretary Thompson's staff, while vetting her nomination, had asked politically motivated questions including whether she would be "an advocate on ergonomics issues."[13] As one person close to this incident put it, taking all the above details into consideration, "I don't know for sure why these respected scientists were kicked out, but it sure smelled foul."[14]

A NEW PLEDGE OF ALLEGIANCE

Like Pamela Kidd, many scientists have come forward with tales of inappropriate, politically motivated questioning by the Bush administration in the appointment process. The February 2004 report *Scientific Integrity in Policymaking: An Investigation into the Bush Administration's Misuse of Science*, released by the Union of Concerned Scientists (UCS), documented several cases in which political litmus tests had been applied by representatives of the Bush administration to candidates for scientific advisory positions.[15]

One such case involved William R. Miller, a distinguished professor of psychology and psychiatry at the University of New Mexico. Miller, who pioneered a leading substance abuse treatment and is the author of more than one hundred articles in peer-reviewed scientific journals, stated that his 2002 interview for a slot on a National Institute on Drug

Abuse advisory panel included questions about whether his views were congruent with those held by President Bush and whether he had voted for Bush in 2000. Presumably based on his answers, Miller said, he was denied the appointment.[16]

In his official response to the UCS report, the Bush administration's science adviser John Marburger called the charges that the administration had used political litmus tests "preposterous." "The UCS asserts that a political litmus test was the reason why Dr. William Miller was denied an appointment on the National Institute on Drug Abuse (NIDA) advisory panel. This claim is false," Marburger wrote. As he explained, the decision to reject Miller was not "based on any conversations with any members of the Secretary's Office [at the Department of Health and Human Services]."[17]

Notably, though, the report had never alleged anything about conversations with any particular Bush administration officials, and specifically not "members of the Secretary's Office." Marburger's strenuous denial carefully avoided the key point: he said nothing about the fact that *some* Bush administration officials had questioned Miller about whom he had voted for.

Since the initial publication of the UCS report in 2004, many more scientists have disclosed their personal experiences with political litmus tests applied by the Bush administration in the appointment process for a wide range of scientific advisory positions. Taken together, their stories suggest a systematic effort to try to empanel only scientists who declare their allegiance to George W. Bush and the Republican Party. The charges, never "preposterous" in the first place, are now so pervasive as to appear indisputable. Yet neither Marburger nor anyone else in the Bush administration has responded to them further.

Consider the experience of Sharon Smith, the chair of the marine biology department at the Rosenstiel School of Marine and Atmospheric Science at the University of Miami. She claims that she was summarily rejected for a position on the U.S. Arctic Research Commission—a presidential appointment—after she gave a less-than-enthusiastic answer in response to a question from the White House personnel office about whether she supported President Bush.

Smith, an arctic ecology expert, had been nominated in 2004 to serve on the Arctic Research Commission, which advises both the White

House and Congress on arctic research issues. She says that, when the White House personnel office called to review her credentials, "The first and only question was, 'Do you support the president?'" As Smith put it: "I was dumbfounded. My first response was that I was not supportive of his foreign and economic policies but that I didn't see what that had to do with my being nominated, or with arctic science. After that, there were no other discussions. I realized the conversation was over.

"Forty years of work in ocean science and you're excluded because you can't say 'I totally support the president of the United States'?" Smith asks incredulously. "I've been on advisory committees before, and I've never had this kind of question. I was outraged."[18]

Further examples of political litmus tests have surfaced from scientists nominated for high-ranking science advisory positions at the National Institutes of Health "council level"; these too merit discussion.

NIH is an enormous family of institutions that serves as steward of medical and behavioral research in the United States. It is divided into some two dozen separate centers and institutes, most of which have a national advisory council or board that serves as the oversight tier of the peer review process—a process upon which the NIH and the entire scientific community relies. Scientists asked to serve on these councils have traditionally been chosen based on their distinguished scientific credentials and technical expertise.

The NIH councils do not set or even recommend policy on behalf of the federal government. Rather, their task is to oversee the process of allocating federal research funds. While their decisions frequently affect the direction of scientific research, this is done based on the merits of proposals submitted and the cumulative expertise of the council members. Because of this vital independent role outside of the policymaking arena, committee heads at NIH have traditionally received wide latitude in determining the scientific expertise needed in their particular area of concern.

It is also worth noting that the law establishing these councils is very clear in its intention to create scientific, not political or policymaking bodies. According to the guidelines published by the Office of Federal Advisory Committee Policy: "The basic criterion for [scientists chosen for] membership on NIH committees is excellence in biomedical and behavioral research. . . . The Federal Advisory Committee Act (FACA), under which NIH committees operate, requires that membership must be fairly balanced in terms of points of view represented and the functions to be performed by the advisory committee."[19]

Under the Bush administration, though, two members appointed to the National Advisory Council for Human Genome Research, Richard Myers of Stanford University and George Weinstock of Baylor College of Medicine, testify that they were each subjected to inappropriate questions about their political views by representatives from the White House during their confirmation process.

Myers, a biochemist, could hardly have had a more distinguished scientific career. He currently holds positions as chair of the Department of Genetics at Stanford University and director of Stanford's Human Genome Center. A recognized expert in genome analysis and the study of DNA variation, his research has furthered worldwide scientific understanding of numerous genetic disorders, including Huntington's disease, progressive myoclonus epilepsy, and basal cell carcinoma.

In the spring of 2002, Myers was notified that he had been nominated to serve on the National Advisory Council for Human Genome Research, an NIH Council-level position. Shortly thereafter, he says, he received a call from Secretary Tommy Thompson's office at HHS.[20] The caller began asking questions about Myers's background and scientific credentials that, he recounts, soon turned increasingly political in nature. First, he recalls, he was asked questions about his view of stem cell research. "I was a little surprised," he says, "given what I know about the nature of the committee's work." (The National Advisory Council for Human Genome Research advises NIH and HHS on genetics, genomic research, training, and programs related to the human genome initiative.) But Myers answered the question candidly. "I told the official that I was in favor of stem cell research. I said that my father has Parkinson's disease and that I would very much like to see a cure. I believe I said it would be a crime in my view if we didn't do that kind of research.

"Then," Myers recalls, "the staffer asked questions that really shocked me. She wanted to know what I thought about President Bush: did I like him, what did I think of the job he was doing." Myers, who describes himself as normally "nonpolitical," objected to the line of questioning. "I said that I thought it was inappropriate to be asked these kinds of questions which led, I think, to an awkward situation for both of us," he says. "She said that she had been told that she needed to ask the questions, and it appeared to me that she was reading from a prepared list. Because of her persistence, I tried to answer in the most nonspecific way possible. I talked about terrorism and the fact that it seemed that the attack of September 11 had brought the country together. But there is no doubt that I felt the questions were an affront and highly inappropriate."

Not long after this interview, Myers was notified that he had been denied the NIH Council position. "I was very depressed," he says. "I really wanted to serve in this capacity. I care deeply about the science, and I'm an expert in this area." Most notably, Myers knew that he had been selected by his NIH colleagues, and so he believed that his rejection must have been because his answers to the political questions posed had been deemed unsatisfactory. Alarmed, he appealed his case directly to Francis Collins, chair of the National Advisory Council for Human Genome Research and director of the branch of NIH called the National Human Genome Research Institute.

Collins declined to be interviewed about the matter. But, through his office, he confirmed the fact that, learning of the circumstances, he personally intervened on Myers behalf to successfully insist that he be allowed to serve on the NIH Council.[21]

Nor is Myers's case an anomaly. His colleague George Weinstock, for instance, tells a remarkably similar story. Weinstock, a microbiologist at Baylor College of Medicine, who was among the appointees to the same NIH advisory panel in 2002, says that he too was subjected to questioning about his political views. Weinstock is also an extremely distinguished researcher, a professor in the departments of molecular and human genetics and molecular virology and microbiology as well as codirector of Baylor's Human Genome Sequencing Center. After learning of his nomination, Weinstock says he received a call from someone at HHS. He too was asked a series of questions that he describes as "leading political questions that had nothing to do with my role on the NIH committee."[22]

Weinstock also reports that the interview included questions about his political views, whether he supported stem cell research, and what he thought of President Bush. "There is no doubt in my mind that these questions represented a political litmus test," he says. He says that while he found the line of questioning disturbing, he chose not to confront the questioner but tried instead "to change the subject. I said things like: 'We live in complicated times.'" As Weinstock puts it, his answers must have been "innocuous enough to be palatable," because he was confirmed by the White House to serve on the NIH Council.

In another instance, Claire Sterk, a current council member at the National Institute on Drug Abuse, states that she too was subjected to repeated questioning about her political views in three separate calls from a White House staff member. Among the questions she was asked, and refused to answer, was whether she had voted for President George W. Bush.

"I have nothing to hide," Sterk commented. "But I told the questioner that I did not see the connection between his line of questioning and my work on a scientific advisory council. And I refused to answer unless the questioner could tell me that I would have some kind of particular political policy role, which I knew I would not." Sterk was confirmed for a position on the NIH Council. She says she believes that, despite her refusal to cooperate, a high-ranking NIH official intervened on behalf of her nomination. Nonetheless, she says she finds it deeply disturbing that the Bush administration would subject its nominees for a scientific advisory position to such intrusive, partisan political questions.[23]

Sterk's dismay is widely shared in the scientific community, where practitioners almost uniformly agree that questions of political affiliation have no place in the confirmation process. And yet, as the stories told here indicate, the practice of subjecting scientists to political litmus tests has become commonplace in the Bush administration. These stories hit a nerve because they represent a kind of overt affront to democratic process that smacks of McCarthy-era blacklists and loyalty pledges.

Most troubling, when politics is injected in such an overt way into the federal government's elaborate system for receiving scientific and technical advice, it threatens to skew the information that policymakers receive. Politically "loyal" advisers may too often tell an administration what it wants to hear or shy away from raising vital concerns in a timely fashion. And at the very least, of course, such politicization means that the nation is denied the advice and counsel of some of its leading experts. As Donald Kennedy, the editor of *Science* and a former president of Stanford University, has commented: "I don't think any administration has penetrated so deeply into the advisory committee structure as this one, and I think it matters. If you start picking people by their ideology instead of their scientific credentials, you are inevitably reducing the quality of the advisory group."[24]

Despite the administration's initial blustering and hapless denial by John Marburger, enough stories like these have surfaced to spur some surprisingly blunt governmental responses. In 2004 two important agencies issued reports explicitly denouncing the use of political litmus tests.

A report from the National Academy of Sciences, released in November 2004, is particularly forceful on the subject. Written by a panel including three former science advisers to both Democratic and Republican administrations, the report unequivocally declares: "It is no more appropriate to ask S&T [Science and Technology] experts to provide nonrelevant information—such as voting record, political-party affiliation, or position on particular policies—than to ask them other personal and immaterial information, such as hair color or height. This type of information has no relevance in discussions related to S&T." As the NAS panel wisely counsels, the nation is best served when scientists for advisory positions are selected "on the basis of their scientific and technical knowledge and credentials and their professional and personal integrity."[25]

So far it is unclear whether, in response to such high-level admonitions, top Bush administration officials will reconsider their political litmus test policy. Should they decide to, one of the indisputable benefits will be that the administration could avoid rejecting candidates on the basis of mistaken identity. That is what happened to William E. Howard III, an engineer from McLean, Virginia. Howard reported in a letter to *Science* that he was told by a member of the Army Science Board (ASB) staff that his nomination to a Defense Department advisory panel was rejected because he had contributed to the presidential campaign of Senator John McCain (R-AZ). In fact, says Howard, he never made such a contribution; instead, as it turns out, someone with a similar name—a William S. Howard—had contributed the money.[26]

BRAVE NEW RULES

The second report on federal litmus tests was issued by the Government Accountability Office (GAO) in April 2004 and politely titled *Federal Ad-*

visory Committees: Additional Guidance Could Help Agencies Better Ensure Independence and Balance. The GAO made twelve specific recommendations to help remove politics from the appointment process to scientific and technical advisory panels. Most of these suggestions call upon branches of the government such as the General Services Administration and the Office of Governmental Ethics to spell out more clearly the guidelines for how the process ought to be handled in the federal government.

The GAO report also astutely notes that even the perception of bias can have a devastating effect. As the report states, when the federal advisory committee system comes to be seen as politicized, it "can jeopardize the value of an individual committee's work; discourage the participation of scientists, experts, and other potential members on future advisory committees; and call into question the integrity of the federal advisory committee system itself."[27]

Sadly, though, the report's message seemed to fall on deaf ears. At the time it appeared, federal officials were dealing with a related situation. The biennial international AIDS meeting was scheduled for July 2004, and the Bush administration was trying to exert political control over which scientists would be allowed to attend. The government had sent 236 government scientists and staff to the previous AIDS meeting in Barcelona, Spain, in 2002. But in the spring of 2004, HHS secretary Tommy Thompson issued a directive that the Bush administration would fund only 50 Americans to attend the upcoming meeting, sidelining scores of scientists who had already had their papers accepted for presentation.

The Bush administration initially explained that the decision was part of a cost-cutting campaign at HHS. But an article in the journal *Science* reported that a confidential email from a high-ranking HHS official sent in March explained that the decision was made "as a result of the treatment [Thompson] received in Barcelona." At that meeting, Thompson had been heckled during a speech by some one hundred activists angry at U.S. funding levels of international AIDS programs. The Bush administration declined to comment on the email.[28]

By June of the same year, the Bush administration dramatically expanded this new strategy to exert political control over access to scientists in the federal government. It announced that all requests from the World Health Organization for U.S. scientists to participate at its meetings would henceforth need to be routed to a political appointee of the administration for review. Previously, U.S. government scientists had made their own arrangements to participate in response to invitations and received approval for travel funds when needed.[29]

This misguided and politically motivated effort to micromanage the schedules of government scientists was lambasted from practically all sides. Perhaps most notable were the objections of D. A. Henderson, a world-renowned epidemiologist who had worked at the World Health Organization for eleven years directing its effort to eradicate smallpox. "I do not feel this is an appropriate or constructive thing to do," he said, adding that science thrives on an "open process." In his experience, Henderson noted, only "small Eastern European countries" had ever required such political permission for their scientists' participation.

What made Henderson's comments particularly potent is his close relationship with the Bush administration. Not only had George W. Bush presented him with the Presidential Medal of Freedom, but Henderson ran the Bush administration's Office of Public Health Preparedness and served as an official adviser to Secretary Thompson. Yet even Henderson's objections did nothing to hamper the policy, which remains in effect to this day.

The sad fact is that, in its efforts to "stack the deck" against scientists and independent technical experts, the Bush administration does not seem to care much about the perception of politicization. And while it has received reprimands for its handling of the process through which scientists are appointed to advisory positions, it has also shown itself to be brazen and creative in its efforts to inject politics into the processes through which scientists and other experts interact with the government and the public.

One such effort currently under way involves governmentwide rule changes proposed by the White House Office of Management and Budget (OMB) that would alter the way the federal government gathers and reviews scientific and technical information. If adopted, the rule changes will have a dramatic effect on the way the government reviews scientific information and promulgates new regulations.

The proposed rules would give the OMB centralized control of the review of scientific information relied upon in policymaking at federal agencies. The most sweeping change would prohibit most scientists and other experts who receive funding from a government agency from serving as peer reviewers, a provision that would sideline vast segments of the academic scientific and technical community. Meanwhile, scientists, engineers, or other experts employed or funded by industry would be permitted to serve as reviewers unless they had a direct financial interest in the issue under review. Clearly, such provisions would dramatically shift the balance in the selection of peer reviewers, giving industry a far greater influence over the flow of scientific and technical information that serves as the basis for formulation of new government regulations.

In response to the dramatic industry handout proposed by the Bush administration, Bruce Alberts, president of the National Academy of Sciences, diplomatically objected that "the highly prescriptive type of peer review that the OMB is proposing differs from accepted practices of peer review in the scientific community, and if enacted in its present form is likely to be counterproductive."[30] Concerned about the impact on the FDA, even the Pharmaceutical Research and Manufacturers of America told the OMB that its proposed rule "would contribute little value and would add to the time and expense of a gatekeeper function that has historically been criticized for obstruction and delay."[31]

As of June 2006, it remains unclear whether the OMB's proposals will become the law of the land. Given the Bush administration's track record on the politicization of scientific and technical information, however, it seems clear that diplomacy and politeness promise little success in curbing the excesses. Thankfully, many individual scientists, health practitioners, and others, as well as scientific and technical associations, have been more forceful in the denunciations of such overt politicization. One such critic is Anthony Robbins, a professor of public health at Tufts University School of Medicine, a co-editor of the *Journal of Public Health Policy,* and the former director of the National Institute for Occupational Safety and Health. The OMB's proposed rule change, Robbins explains plainly, threatens to "radically restrict access to scientific advice at the government agencies on which we rely to protect public health. The White House could restrict open discussion and tilt the balance of residual discussions towards commercial interests.

"In the hands of the Bush administration," Robbins warns, "these could be the tools that could ultimately destroy integrity in science as we know it."[32]

9

Stem Cells and Monkey Trials

> When prominent scientists must fear that descriptions of their research will be misrepresented and misused by their government to advance political ends, something is deeply wrong.
>
> ELIZABETH BLACKBURN, microbiologist, University of California,
> San Francisco, Medical School, April 2004

George W. Bush campaigned as someone who would work well with people of different perspectives and political persuasions. "I showed the people of Texas that I'm a uniter, not a divider," Bush famously told the conservative journalist and commentator David Horowitz back in 1999. "I refuse to play the politics of putting people into groups and pitting one group against another."[1]

The reality, of course, is that the two terms of the George W. Bush presidency have exhibited a virtually unprecedented level of partisanship. The Bush administration has, time and again, allowed political considerations to distort the government's handling of information about even the most critical matters of national security, environmental safety, and public health. This proclivity for allowing ideology to trump fact-based data and analysis plays into the administration's willingness to pander to minority factions at the expense of the public interest. The resulting ideologically motivated postures have frequently placed the administration at odds with the scientists and technical experts in the federal government who are trained to revere the powerful role data can play in guiding policymaking.

Yet even these frequent clashes over factual data fall short of capturing Bush's apparent antipathy to the nation's scientific and technological elite. One of the most remarkable features of the George W. Bush presidency is the way he has so often seemed to go out of his way to antago-nize the scientific community. For example, there was the combination of a long delay in appointing his science adviser, John Marburger III, and the simultaneous demotion of the science adviser post. Or the fact that Bush appointed a nonscientist, Richard Russell, to serve as Marburger's associate director at the Office of Science and Technology Policy. It was the first time in memory that the post—which has broad responsibility over the way science and technology issues are handled by the federal government—had been held by anyone who wasn't a credentialed sci-entist.[2] In his relationship with the scientific community, there is little question that Bush has been a "divider."

A telling case in point is the administration's dismissal of Elizabeth Blackburn, one of the nation's top scientists, in February 2004. Sixty of the nation's most prominent scientists had just released their well-publicized "scientists' statement" questioning the Bush administration's scientific integrity. And the Union of Concerned Scientists had issued the accompanying report, *Scientific Integrity in Policymaking,* upon which this book is based. The topic of the Bush administration's lack of scien-tific integrity was in the headlines and on the airwaves daily. At the height of this public attention, President Bush chose to alter the compo-sition of his Presidential Advisory Council on Bioethics.

On February 27, 2004, the White House personnel office told Eliza-beth Blackburn, a leading cell biologist, and William May, a prominent medical ethicist, that their appointments to the bioethics council would not be renewed. The timing made a decisive statement indeed, for Black-burn and May had frequently disagreed with the administration's posi-tions on the ethics of biomedical research.[3] In particular, they had dis-sented regarding the Bush administration's policy of limiting government funding for stem cell research. Even more significant, though, was the symbolism of the Bush administration's move, especially with regard to Blackburn. In ousting her, Bush was dismissing one of the foremost ex-perts in her field.

Blackburn is best known as the co-discoverer of telomerase, an en-zyme linked to cancer cell growth. The discovery launched an entire field of cancer research. The Nobel laureate Tom Cech, the president of Howard Hughes Medical Institute, spoke for many when he described

Blackburn as not only "very smart and successful," but as "one of the top biomedical researchers in the world."[4]

Scientists take their accolades seriously, and there are few that Blackburn has yet to receive. She is a member of the National Institute of Medicine and the National Academy of Sciences and a fellow of the American Academy of Arts and Sciences, the American Association for the Advancement of Science, and the Royal Society of London. She is also the past president of the American Society for Cell Biology (ASCB), which represents eleven thousand scientists worldwide.[5] So it was no surprise that the ASCB issued a public statement charging that Blackburn's dismissal reflected a pattern in the Bush administration in which politics trumps science. Harvey Lodish, then president of the normally apolitical ASCB, excoriated the Bush administration for a move he said would "significantly undermine the ability of the Council" to base its considerations on a scientific foundation.[6]

As Blackburn herself pointed out, at the time of her dismissal, she was one of only three full-time biomedical scientists on the seventeen-person panel, so that it was already weighted heavily to nonscientists with strong ideological views. Of course, no one disputes that nonscientists can and should play an important role on a bioethics panel. But most would also agree that scientists should be represented on a panel charged with considering biomedical issues.

As the incident unfolded, Blackburn claimed that she was dismissed because she disapproved of the Bush administration's highly restrictive position on stem cell research. In fact, she said, her dismissal had come soon after she objected to a council report on stem cell research. In an essay in the *New England Journal of Medicine* in April 2004, Blackburn revealed that her point of view, which she believes reflects the scientific consensus in America, was not included in the council's reports even though those reports were supposed to present the views of all the council's members.[7]

The council chair, Leon Kass, publicly disputed Blackburn's charges.[8] But the Bush administration had no answer to the obvious fact that the removal of Blackburn and May significantly limited the range of views available to the president on bioethics issues. This was because the administration replaced Blackburn and May (as well as one other panel member who had previously resigned) with three appointees known pri-marily for their ideological positions on stem cell research. The new ap-pointees included Ben Carson, a pediatric neurosurgeon at Johns Hop-kins Medical Center, who had championed the importance of religious values in public life; Peter Lawler, a political philosopher, who had pub-licly praised Kass's work; and Diana Schaub, a political scientist, who had described as "evil" any research in which embryos are destroyed.[9]

The Bush administration's relationship with the scientific community had been strained prior to this incident. But the decision to dismiss Black-burn sent a clear signal: if the nation's top scientists questioned his sci-entific integrity, Bush seemed to be saying, he would simply show that he had little use for their advice anyway.

Not surprisingly, the incident made the rift between the Bush admin-istration and the scientific community more public than ever. In the wake of Blackburn's dismissal, some 170 researchers signed an open letter to President Bush protesting the decision.[10] So did some twenty-seven Dem-ocratic U.S. senators, including then Senate minority leader Tom Daschle. As the senators put it: "Only days after the [Union of Con-cerned Scientists] report's release, your administration added another shameful example of the deception and distortion that the report docu-ments."[11] One of the remaining biomedical members of the bioethics panel—Janet Rowley, a medical professor at the University of Chicago—may have best summed up the situation. Blackburn's dismissal, Rowley said, was "an important example of the absolutely destructive practices of the Bush administration."[12]

STEM CELL DECREE

Of course, George W. Bush's strained relationship with the scientific community began long before the Blackburn saga. Things began to sour, in fact, with Bush's first major policy announcement in 2001: an edict limiting federal funding for embryonic stem cell research. It is worth looking closely at this stem cell decision, not just because of its vital im-portance to the scientific community and human health in the future, but for what it shows about Bush's decision-making process on such a com-plex matter.

First, let's review some of the science involved.

Since embryonic stem cells first began to be studied in mice, spawning a literal revolution in developmental biology in the 1980s, they have been the subject of tremendous interest and excitement among biomedical researchers worldwide. The cells are derived from the inner cell mass of what scientists call *blastocysts*—a stage of embryo development reached roughly five to nine days after fertilization. What makes these embryonic cells so exciting to researchers is that they are "pluripotent," which means they have the potential to turn into any cell in the body. They are also continually self-replicating so, if perpetuated in the lab, a so-called cell line of embryonic stem cells can offer a theoretically endless supply of such cells.[13] Because of the pluripotency of these cells, scientists believe that human embryonic stem cells may one day serve as a kind of toolkit that could be directed, when injected into the body, to treat diseases from diabetes to muscular dystrophy.

To the extent that controversy exists about human embryonic stem cells—and it does at least in the mind of George W. Bush—it derives from the fact that, as currently practiced, the process of retrieving them requires the destruction of the blastocysts they come from, that is, from fertilized human eggs.

Biomedical technology that manipulates human cells certainly raises important ethical and moral questions. But even if you believe that human life is formed at the moment of conception, blastocysts put such a religious conviction to a severe test. A blastocyst is about as wide as a single human hair: a tiny clump of some two hundred cells that, when seen under the microscope, displays no remotely recognizable human features. In fact, at this stage, it is still possible for a blastocyst to divide to become a set of identical twins—which in and of itself makes it dubious to think of a blastocyst as an individual human life.[14]

It is also worth making two additional points about blastocysts. The first is that their destruction is a natural human commonplace. According to scientists' best estimates, as many as 80 percent of the blastocysts created by human sexual intercourse never make it to term, either failing to implant in the uterus or otherwise self-destructing.[15] The second is that, thanks to the popularity of in-vitro fertilization (IVF), which has reportedly resulted so far in more than 250,000 births in the United States,[16] there are many unwanted blastocysts on hand. One study estimates, for instance, that more than 400,000 are currently stored in freezers at in-vitro fertilization clinics across the country. The vast majority of these are held for a certain time in case couples who have used IVF want to try to further enlarge their families, but are eventually discarded. At least 11,000 blastocysts have been specifically designated for research by the couples that created them.[17]

Stem cells have, for years, received a good deal of discussion in the press as a medical marvel. But the public first learned of President Bush's policy on embryonic stem cell research on August 9, 2001, when he went on television from his ranch in Texas to announce it.[18] "I have given this issue a great deal of thought, prayer, and considerable reflection," Bush told the nation. He also invoked the unnerving red herring of Aldous Huxley's *Brave New World,* with its vision of human babies born in factories. Noting that he believed "human life is a sacred gift from our Creator," Bush made what the administration later tried to portray as a Solomonic decision to terminate federal funding for all *new* embryonic stem cell lines while allowing the federal government to continue to fund researchers using those cell lines that already existed as of that particular August evening.

In his address, President Bush said that "60 genetically diverse stem cell lines" were available for such use by scientists. But, as Stephen Hall has noted in the *New York Times,* the number "was a fiction," resulting from the lack of competent advice on the topic.[19] Despite Bush's self-proclaimed "reflection" on the matter, it is noteworthy how little scientific advice he had actually received. The occasion of such an important policy on biomedical research would have been the perfect opportunity for Bush to consult with the administration's science adviser, for instance. But, as we have seen, some six months into the administration, Bush and his team had still not bothered to send the Senate a nominee for the post.[20]

In fact, the true number of available stem cell lines was a fraction of the number Bush claimed, and even those were of questionable utility for any clinically useful human treatment. As we now know, Bush's claim resulted from the fact that, a week before his address, a delegation from the National Institutes of Health had informed the president and his advisers that approximately sixty so-called *derivations* of human embryonic stem cells existed.[21] The distinction between a derivation and a cell line was a crucial one because, until scientists are actually able to sustain the growth of the cells in culture, they have no idea whether they will succeed as viable cell lines that can be used in research and shared with other laboratories.

As the Nobel laureate and emeritus Stanford medical professor Paul Berg later colorfully explained, the existence of the derivations simply meant that, on sixty different occasions, "somebody took a blastocyst from an IVF clinic and cracked it open and poured everything into a vial and stuck it into a liquid nitrogen tank—in which case we don't know if it's a line. And most of them died, and that's why there are so few now."[22]

According to Stephen Hall, the same day President Bush learned of the sixty embryonic cell derivations, he subsequently met with the bioethicist LeRoy Walters of Georgetown University, who expressed his skepticism that so many viable cell lines were available.[23] So it seems the distinction between viable cell lines and derivations was already either misunderstood or conveniently ignored by Bush.

Despite Walters's warning, President Bush persisted in his fallacy about the number of existing embryonic cell lines. He either spoke to so few experts in the field that it was never brought forcefully enough to his attention, or, at least as likely, he simply chose the number that made his edict seem more palatable, offering the illusion that scientific research need not be significantly impeded. Either way, the prospect is disheartening, to say the least.

Of course, after Bush's announcement, scientists at the National Institutes of Health and elsewhere instantly realized the president's mistake. Researchers around the country immediately challenged his numbers.[24] In now-familiar fashion, though, despite the outcry from the scientific community, the Bush administration clung steadfastly to its claim about the number of available cell lines. The absurd national "debate" that ensued was, after all, a question of discernible fact. It reached something of a crescendo when, after a month of relentless criticism in the Senate and elsewhere, Secretary of Health and Human Services Tommy Thompson admitted that only some two dozen embryonic stem cell lines were available.[25]

In the aftermath of Thompson's admission, the scientific community was finally making headway in its case that the number of stem cell lines permitted for federal funding by the Bush administration was far too small to support a robust research effort. But then the terrorist attacks of September 11, 2001, understandably eclipsed the subject. Later that month, with little public notice, the National Institutes of Health amended the nation's registry of embryonic cell lines. At that time, when all was said and done, there were, as a result of the Bush edict, just nine cell lines known to be usable that were available to U.S.-funded scientists by the government's official count.[26]

The main point, of course, is not how many cell lines President Bush actually sanctioned—researchers now call them "the presidential lines"—but that he considered the matter so superficially that he got this central fact badly wrong. And even if he had been accurate about the paltry number of cell lines he was permitting, his embryonic stem cell policy would still stand as an embarrassment, a fiasco, and an outrage. The Bush stem cell edict is arbitrary and morally inconsistent. It is overwhelmingly disapproved of by the American public, even, polls say, by a majority of Republicans.[27] Over the past four years, states (including the biotech powerhouses California and Massachusetts) and private institutions have been forced to try to fill the breach by offering a hospitable climate and much-needed funding for stem cell researchers.[28] The U.S. House has voted to overturn Bush's stem cell policy, and, as of this writing, the Senate is poised to do the same.[29] And yet Bush has vowed to veto this legislative effort in order to retain his edict. If he should follow through, it would be the first veto in his six years in office.

One of the many ironies about the Bush policy is that even the president's hand-selected and controversial Bioethics Council—of Elizabeth Blackburn fame—has pointed up its inconsistency. The council's 2004 report *Monitoring Stem Cell Research* (despite Blackburn's assertion that it did not include her views) offers a painstakingly evenhanded review of the moral issues involved—and in the process highlights the glaring problems with the president's edict.[30]

For one thing, as the report discusses, Bush's "line in the sand" on embryonic stem cell research is utterly arbitrary. Why, for instance, did Bush decide it should go into immediate effect? Almost any other leader would have, at the very least, gathered a group of stakeholders together to hammer out the logistics. After all, as noted above, one prominent study estimates that there are some 11,000 unwanted frozen embryos that have been specifically donated for research. Conservatively speaking, scientists say those blastocysts alone could yield at least 275 additional embryonic stem cell lines.[31] Why couldn't Bush have sanctioned the use of those lines since they had already been designated for research purposes prior to his decree?

Such a distinction would have made a world of difference to scientists in the United States. Researchers agree it is unlikely that therapies can be derived from any of the so-called presidential cell lines, because, when human embryonic stem cells were first extracted in the late 1990s, they were often kept alive using "feeder cells" from mice. The practice is perfectly acceptable for studying the cells in the lab but not for clinical uses: it risks the possibility of introducing mouse viruses into humans. More recently, scientists have overcome this problem by growing embryonic stem cell lines uncontaminated by any animal materials. Because of Bush's policy, however, U.S. scientists are not eligible to use federal funding to work on these uncontaminated lines.[32]

The same restrictions curtail U.S.-funded scientists from using the promising technique called "therapeutic cloning" in which the nucleus of a body cell from a person suffering from a given disease is implanted in an unfertilized egg. When the egg begins to divide, scientists can then extract an embryonic stem cell line in which the disease and its development can be closely studied.[33] Under the Bush administration's stem cell regime, however, U.S.-funded scientists are prevented from conducting this research with federal funds: not only are such cells not represented in the presidential lines, but such lines could never result from the process of in-vitro fertilization, the only source Bush sanctioned in even a limited way.

Finally, the Bush edict on stem cells is not only arbitrary but also morally inconsistent. As Bush's own bioethics council notes clearly, morally speaking there can be no middle ground on the issue.[34] If Bush truly likens the destruction of five-day-old blastocysts to the killing of a human being, how can he remain silent about privately funded stem cell research, or for that matter, in-vitro fertilization itself, which is responsible for the nation's vast storehouses of blastocysts in the first place?

It comes as no surprise that such nuance is lost on the Bush administration. In this case, as in so many others, Bush followed "his gut," as he likes to say, letting his personal beliefs dictate policy for the nation. And once he has set his personal moral compass on an issue, Bush famously brooks no deviation, regardless of how many inconvenient facts arise to contradict it. If Bush's bioethics council raises the inconsistencies of his policy, for instance, his solution—rather than grappling with the problems—is to quell the dissent by firing the messenger and empanelling members more predisposed to accept his views.

The sad result of Bush's policy on embryonic stem cells has been to imperil the leadership position of the United States in a vital new area of biomedical research. As George Daley, a stem cell researcher at Harvard Medical School, explained in a recent article in the *New England Journal of Medicine:* "The President's policy has severely curtailed opportunities for U.S. scientists to study the cell lines that have since been established, many of which have unique attributes or represent invaluable models of human disease." Some 128 new human embryonic stem cell lines have been produced worldwide since Bush's announcement, some offering particularly dramatic new possibilities. "Many opportunities are being missed," Daley writes. "The science of human embryonic stem cells is in its infancy, and the current policies threaten to starve the field at a critical stage."[35]

Daley's view is almost universally held among biomedical researchers. Some have responded by trying to continue their research with private funds. At Harvard University, for instance, the stem cell researcher Douglas Melton announced in March 2004 the creation of seventeen new embryonic stem cell lines, supported in part by a grant from the Juvenile Diabetes Research Foundation.[36] Melton has offered to share these cell lines freely with scientists around the world, but, of course, U.S. scientists are permitted to work on them only if they, like Melton, are able to attract the requisite private funding. Most recently, Melton and his colleagues Chad Cowan, Jocelyn Atienza, and Kevin Eggan at Harvard's Stem Cell Institute reported preliminary results on a technique called cell fusion that showed promise in "reprogramming" adult cells to behave like embryonic stem cells.[37] The research is particularly interesting because it could, potentially, offer a technological "end run" around Bush's policy by creating usable stem cells without the need to destroy a blastocyst.

But even with efforts like these, there is no escaping the fact that Bush's edict has slowed the development of one of the most promising areas of biomedical research—a field that might someday help treat millions with a wide range of diseases. And this decision continues to draw criticism from most researchers in the field.

By May 2005, following the passage of legislation in the U.S. House of Representatives to undo President Bush's restrictions on stem cell research, dissent about the president's policy even surfaced for the first time from within the Bush administration, when the views of several directors of the National Institutes of Health—all Bush appointees—were publicly released. Elizabeth Nabel, director of the National Heart, Lung, and Blood Institute, stated: "Progress has been delayed by the limited number of cell lines. The NIH has ceded leadership in this field."[38] Nora D. Volkow, director of the National Institute on Drug Abuse, complained that access to the few approved lines of stem cells is "complicated and expensive."[39] James Battey, the head of stem cell research at NIH, worried aloud that some of the best stem cell biologists would leave NIH as a result of Bush's policy.[40]

Why hadn't the public learned earlier about the views of these prominent government scientists? As one political commentator put it: "Because their politically appointed masters at the Department of Health and Human Services had kept them muzzled." In fact, the views of these top NIH scientists had come to light under telling and unusual circumstances. Senator Arlen Specter (R-PA), an opponent of Bush's stem cell policy, bypassed normal procedure to solicit candid assessments on behalf of the Senate Subcommittee on Labor, Health and Human Services and Education. As Senator Specter specifically directed these top government scientists: "Your response should be submitted directly to the Subcommittee *without editing, revision, or comment by the Department of Health and Human Services*" (emphasis added).[41]

BUSH'S NEW "MONKEY TRIAL"

We have reviewed the Bush administration's repeated denials of fact on a wide array of topics from national security to public health. We have seen an administration that stubbornly insisted that Iraq's aluminum tubes were for the enrichment of uranium when technical analysis indicated otherwise; that global warming remains in doubt when plainly it doesn't; that abstinence-only programs will reduce the prevalence of sexually transmitted diseases when, by themselves, they will almost surely do the opposite. So perhaps it should come as no surprise that George W. Bush, in the summer of 2005, shared with the nation his doubts about evolution, surely the most overdetermined, fact-based pillar of modern biology.

This latest affront to the scientific community came during a question-and-answer session with a small group of Texas reporters at the White House, in which Bush endorsed the idea that creationism in its latest guise—known as "intelligent design"—ought to be taught alongside evolution in the nation's schools.

Did Bush really think American children in the twenty-first century should be taught a religious "alternative" to evolution in science class?

"I think that part of education is to expose people to different schools of thought," the president said. "You're asking me whether or not people ought to be exposed to different ideas; the answer is yes."[42] Bush's comment was wrapped in the veil of "tolerance for different viewpoints" that is one of the clever ploys of the intelligent design movement. But that does not obscure the profoundly anti-science nature of this statement.

After all, the viewpoint championed by Bush is not some new, emerging challenge to evolution but itself a direct evolutionary descendant of the creationism that has railed against Darwin's theory ever since *On the Origin of Species* was published nearly 150 years ago. Then as now creationists, as Christian literalists, take issue with evolution for not comporting with the Bible's book of Genesis. As more than a century of wrangling has already shown, a fact-based debate of the issue cannot resolve the matter because such strict fundamentalists have little use for the facts of natural science. Their view is based in a literal acceptance of the validity of what is told in the Bible. According to the Bible's teachings, for instance, the earth's age is determined not by measuring the decay of long-lived radioisotopes, for instance, but by counting back the number of generations the Bible lists as having descended from Adam and Eve.

Because an ecumenical sense of religious freedom is one of the fundamental tenets of U.S. democracy, people are free to believe whatever they wish as a matter of religious faith. Along these lines, it would be one thing for Bush to have exhorted children in the United States to study the Bible. It is quite another matter, however, to offer up the Bible as a reasonable "alternative" to empirically based science. But that is exactly what Bush did. It is what proponents of the intelligent design movement explicitly call for.

True, in this latest creationist variant, advocates of so-called intelligent design don't speak much about the Bible. Backed by a multi-million-dollar Christian Right think tank in Seattle called the Discovery Institute, they use more slick, pseudoscientific language.[43] They talk about things like "irreducible complexity." The argument goes like this: organs such as the human eye are too complicated and have too many intricately interlinking parts to have evolved over millennia; therefore, they exhibit the hand of an "intelligent designer."[44]

Some have noted that, with its toned-down references to religion, intelligent design actually represents a retreat on the part of creationists because, to the chagrin of many Christian fundamentalists, the movement does concede some aspects of evolution. As one of the movement's main textbooks puts it, "The idea of intelligent design does not preclude the possibility that variation within species occurs, or that new species are formed from existing populations."[45] The passage is not lost on Eugenie Scott, executive director of the National Center for Science Education in Oakland, California, a nonprofit group that monitors attacks on the teaching of evolution. As Scott quipped recently: "You have to hand it to the creationists. They have evolved."[46]

But while the rhetoric may have softened, intelligent design has not altered the creationist goal of undermining on essentially religious grounds the teaching of evolution in the classroom. It has merely adapted to the fact that U.S. courts have prohibited overtly religious creationist views from being taught in the nation's public school system. As one eloquently worded 1982 court verdict put it: "No group, no matter how large or small, may use the organs of government, of which the public schools are the most conspicuous and influential, to foist its religious beliefs on others."[47]

Of course, in the age-old battles over evolution whose embers President Bush stoked with his comments, the best-known American skirmish occurred in the 1925 Scopes "Monkey Trial." Thanks in large part to the 1960 Hollywood version, *Inherit the Wind,* in which Spencer Tracy masterfully played the fictionalized version of Scopes's lawyer, Clarence Darrow, many people believe that the trial decisively settled the issue of teaching evolution in school. Unfortunately, the real story didn't work out that way. In the real case, John Scopes, a high school teacher, was convicted of having violated Tennessee's Butler Act, which, like many states' creationist laws, explicitly prohibited teaching evolution, or "any theory that denies the Story of Divine Creation of Man as taught in the Bible."[48] Scopes's conviction was then overturned on a technicality, so he never even had the chance to challenge the constitutionality of the Butler Act on appeal. Astonishingly, the anti-evolution law remained in effect in Tennessee until 1968 when it was struck down by the Supreme Court.[49]

Thanks to the resourceful persistence of the creationists, the legal battles have continued despite the Supreme Court verdict. Creationists in Arkansas notoriously tried to put an anti-evolution law on the books in 1981, but the effort was struck down in the 1982 court decision cited above. And the battles continue to this day. The recently decided case *Kitzmiller et al. v. Dover Area School District et al.*, in Harrisburg, Pennsylvania, struck down the Dover school district's rule that teachers must read a disclaimer when they teach evolution that claims it represents "a theory" and that "gaps in the theory exist for which there is no evidence."[50] Even more recently, emboldened by Bush's remarks, a group of parochial high schools in California has brought a lawsuit challenging the University of California's admission policy of refusing to certify high school science courses that use textbooks challenging Darwin's theory of evolution.[51]

Against this backdrop came President Bush's comments in August 2005, likely unscripted but not accidental. They could not more perfectly encapsulate his hostile relationship to science. Not long after the president's remarks, a "debate" over evolution appeared on the cover of *Time* magazine—and Bush had created his own national "monkey trial" in the court of public opinion.

Needless to say, Bush's remarks earned him few admirers in the scientific community. Even John Marburger, Bush's normally loyal scientific adviser, disavowed the president's comment. "Intelligent design is not a scientific concept," Marburger said, much to his credit, adding that "evolution is the cornerstone of modern biology."[52]

Bush presumably does not care that intelligent design is discredited by the vast majority of the scientific community. But the fact is that, literally and figuratively, evolution is built upon rock-solid evidence. In the

150 years since Darwin's day, a huge number of new findings have been made in the fossil record, which has been pored over meticulously by generations of paleontologists. All this evidence supports evolution.

Similarly, biologists have now observed hundreds of cases of natural selection firsthand. They have closely tracked it, for instance, when bacteria develop resistance to antibiotics; and it is the reason for current fears that a strain of the avian flu virus will mutate to become infectious between humans. Scientists using mitochondrial DNA—a set of genes that is passed directly from a mother to her offspring—for instance, have even traced the human lineage back 150,000 years, tracking the mitochondrial DNA's genetic mutations along the way.[53]

In addition, evolution wins the day against creationist claims on the prevalence of vestigial biological traits alone. Creationists have often cited the case of whales as a species that evolution cannot easily explain.[54] But Jerry Coyne, a professor of evolution at the University of Chicago, notes that, in the last decade, paleontologists have uncovered a nearly complete evolutionary series of whales, beginning with fully terrestrial animals and documenting how descendants became more and more aquatic over time. Using these fossils, researchers have been able to trace the way front limbs evolved into flippers and hind limbs and pelvis were gradually reduced to tiny but still visible vestiges.

"Insofar as intelligent-design theory can be tested scientifically, it has been falsified," Coyne writes. With the widespread prevalence of vestigial organs and other body parts, "organisms simply do not look as if they had been intelligently designed." A good example, Coyne says, is the human appendix, which as he puts it, "is simply a bad thing to have. It is certainly not the product of intelligent design: how many humans died of appendicitis before surgery was invented?"[55]

As the Oxford biologist Richard Dawkins has noted, "Evolution by natural selection is a brilliant answer to the riddle of complexity because it is not a theory of chance. It is a theory of gradual, incremental change over millions of years, which starts with something very simple and works up along slow, gradual gradients to great complexity." Nothing else comes close, he says, to offering an explanation for what we see in the biological world.[56]

And indeed in the scientific community the issue was settled long ago. Proponents of intelligent design make much of purported gaps in what they like to emphasize is "the theory" of evolution. But few conceptual gaps really remain, and evolution is so well substantiated as to be almost universally considered a scientific fact.

Proponents of intelligent design, claiming that they want equal time to "teach the controversy," like to portray evolution as "just" a theory clung to by some closed-minded scientific orthodoxy. But the truth is precisely the opposite. There is no serious controversy because evolution is built upon facts—testable facts—to the best of our ability to discern them. And the work of scientists, as Karl Popper put it so well in *The Logic of Scientific Discovery,* is not to uphold one another's work but to try as hard as possible to falsify it. And despite popular—and creation-ist—usage, this is exactly what "theory" means in science. That is why it is so essential for scientists to try to strip away their preconceptions—faith-based or otherwise—to challenge one another's hypotheses through the peer review process. Through this process, they have shown time and again that they can achieve a fuller and more detailed understanding of how the world works.

Put another way, as the philosopher and historian of science Philip Kitcher explains in his classic work on creationism *Abusing Science,* "scientific theories earn our acceptance by making successful predictions."[57] The intelligent design movement fails to meet this hurdle because it is not testable. It lacks any real evidence. It offers virtually no explanations or peer-reviewed papers in the scientific literature. In this sense, there is really nothing new here since Darwin's day, when his colleague Herbert Spencer, the Victorian-era British biologist and philosopher, famously stated in an 1852 essay: "Those who cavalierly reject the theory of evolution as not adequately supported by facts, seem quite to forget that their own theory is supported by no facts at all."[58]

What can anyone say about a president of the United States who pitches his tent on such untenable ground? After all, the United States is a nation built on science and technology and world renowned for its contributions in these disciplines. Some of the nation's founders, including Benjamin Franklin and Thomas Jefferson, were scientists themselves. The idea of "promoting science and the useful arts" by allowing practitioners to patent their useful inventions is written into the first article of the U.S. Constitution.

Bush's endorsement of bringing "intelligent design" into the classroom was such a stunning repudiation of science that perhaps the best commentary was a pitch-perfect spoof in the weekly *The Onion*. As the "report" began:

> Scientists from the Evangelical Center for Faith-Based Reasoning are now asserting that the long-held "theory of gravity" is flawed, and they have responded to it with a new theory of Intelligent Falling.
>
> "Things fall not because they are acted upon by some gravitational force, but because a higher intelligence, 'God' if you will, is pushing them down," said Gabriel Burdett, who holds degrees in education, applied Scripture, and physics from Oral Roberts University.[59]

The satire succeeds so well because it goes to the heart of the folly at hand. When science detaches itself from facts—that is, from the power of empirical observation—it ceases any longer to be science. As Douglas H. Erwin, a paleobiologist at the Smithsonian, has observed: "One of the rules of science is: no miracles allowed. That's a fundamental presumption of what we do."[60]

In the end, though, despite the pseudoscientific patina, intelligent design is not really about science or facts. Most likely, its roots derive not just from religious fundamentalism but from the deep-seated fear that, evolutionarily speaking, we humans may be closer to the savannah than most of us feel comfortable admitting. In particular, many people seem to fear that, if evolution is true, it somehow deflates our sense of moral purpose as humans—the fervent hope that many hold that we might be the special pinnacle of God's earthly creations. Ultimately, perhaps, the real underlying fear is that our acceptance of the science of evolution will foster an erosion of the Judeo-Christian moral values that so many Americans cherish.

Quite apart from the science, that is why, symbolically, President Bush failed the nation so badly in his comments supporting intelligent design. Had Bush been any kind of statesman, he could easily have tried to reconcile the deep-seated religious qualms about evolution without denigrating the science involved. He could have noted that accepting testable facts about the world does not mean we have to relinquish our moral reasoning. He could have told the nation that the teaching of science need not diminish any moral or spiritual values.

Many scientists hold deep-seated religious beliefs. But no credible scientist believes religion should be injected into an observation and fact-based study of how the world works, from test tubes to telescopes. The idea is profoundly antithetical to the entire scientific enterprise. This central tenet, much like the principle of free speech, or freedom of religion, is not something cast aside lightly. Yet, in his ill-considered, inarticulate, and passing reference to evolution, Bush managed to trample this central tenet that science should remain free of political or religious interference.

In its symbolism, Bush's off-handed comments to reporters perfectly summed up his administration's ongoing and concerted effort to undermine science. His statement demonstrated his profound antipathy for the scientific enterprise: its reliance on higher learning and its insistence on fact-based evidence. Equally troubling, Bush also showed his true colors as a reckless "divider" after all: a demagogue displaying a thoroughly antidemocratic willingness to impose his own sectarian religious views on a pluralistic nation. In so doing, George W. Bush betrayed not just deeply held tenets of science, but tenets of democracy as well.

10

Restoring Scientific Integrity

> We are each entitled to our own opinion, but no one is entitled to his own facts.
>
> DANIEL PATRICK MOYNIHAN, U.S. senator (D-NY), 1977–2001

One of the saddest consequences of the Bush administration's lack of scientific integrity is the large number of dedicated federal officials who have felt driven out of government service.

A good example is Bruce Buckheit, whom we met in chapter 5. Buckheit retired in December 2003 as director of the Air Enforcement Division of the Environmental Protection Agency (EPA) after holding major federal environmental posts for two decades. Since 1997, Buckheit had investigated and ultimately built an enforcement case against some of the nation's largest polluters—coal-fired power plants. As we saw, Buckheit's aim was to get these polluting plants to obey the Clean Air Act's so-called New Source Review provisions. "I came into government with Nixon and Ford," he says. "I'm not politically active, and I always tried to be a good bureaucrat."[1] But when Buckheit realized Bush administration officials were gutting the rules and undermining his agency's efforts to enforce the law, he decided he could not compromise his personal integrity and chose to resign.

Buckheit was not alone in his decision. Many of his colleagues at EPA have felt compelled to do the same.

Richard Biondi, Buckheit's assistant in the Air Enforcement Division, left the agency as well. "We would have stayed," Biondi said, "but we couldn't make the contribution we had initially hoped to make."[2] By the time Buckheit and Biondi resigned from EPA, their boss, Eric Schaeffer, former head of the Office of Regulatory Enforcement, had already quit. In his letter of resignation in February 2002, Schaeffer lamented: "We seem about to snatch defeat from the jaws of victory, fighting a White House that seems determined to weaken the rules we are trying to enforce."[3]

The rules the Bush administration sought to undermine are, of course, provisions of U.S. federal law—hard-won environmental protections of the Clean Air Act that benefit public health and are overwhelmingly favored by Republicans and Democrats alike.

After Schaeffer's resignation, Sylvia Lowrance became EPA's top enforcement official. But just six months later, in August 2002, she chose to resign as well. She had been at the agency for twenty-four years. Like so many career government professionals, Lowrance was loath to publicly criticize the U.S. government or in any way disparage her colleagues who remained at the agency. "I think this many senior people leaving is telling," was all she said to the press.[4]

The Bush administration then appointed J. P. Suarez to head the EPA's enforcement office. He was widely viewed as a loyal Republican Bush appointee; when he resigned in January 2004, he initially followed Bush administration protocol by claiming that his decision to leave had nothing to do with administration policies. But Suarez broke his silence in October 2004, when he told the *Environmental Law Reporter* that the Bush administration had waged "an unforgiving assault" on the EPA's enforcement program. "It became clear to me during my tenure at EPA," Suarez said, that the goal of the Bush administration's reform of New Source Review provisions "was to prevent any enforcement case from going forward." The Bush administration's method, as we have seen in detail, was to manipulate and suppress scientific data and to subvert existing laws through bureaucratic maneuvers. As Suarez put it: "It becomes very difficult when you feel that the people who are your colleagues do not believe in you or your mission."[5]

The loss of so many experienced public servants—Republicans and Democrats alike—is disheartening, to say the least. It also greatly complicates the task of trying to restore and rebuild scientific integrity in federal government processes. Most of the staff members in EPA's enforcement division are lawyers by training. But similar stories abound at the

Centers for Disease Control, the Climate Change Science Program, the Fish and Wildlife Service, the Department of Agriculture, and many other agencies where scientists and other officials collect and evaluate technical information that serves as the basis for government decision making.

Most recently, in August 2005, as discussed in chapter 4, Susan Wood, director of the Office of Women's Health at the Food and Drug Administration, joined the ranks of government officials who have resigned in protest. Wood was outraged by her agency's decision to indefinitely prohibit over-the-counter availability of the emergency contraceptive drug Plan B. "I can no longer serve as staff," she said, "when scientific and clinical evidence, fully evaluated and recommended for approval by the professional staff here, has been overruled."[6]

Buckheit, Biondi, Schaeffer, Suarez, and Wood all aptly convey the demoralization that occurs when government information is not handled with honesty and integrity; when agency reports are suppressed or distorted; and when the government's own experts are shut out of a profoundly undemocratic decision-making process. In these ways, the Bush administration has systematically abused the integrity of U.S. governmental processes. Time and again, Bush administration officials have allowed ideological concerns to trump the evidence-based information compiled by the government's own scientists and expert staff as well as by peer-reviewed scientists and technical experts under government contract. They have also bypassed or subverted accepted governmental processes to push through an ideologically driven policy agenda.

Responding to the ongoing barrage of reports of such abuses and the loss of so many principled federal officials, some in government have proposed legislative and bureaucratic remedies. As discussed in chapter 8, both the National Academy of Sciences and the Government Accountability Office released reports offering specific recommendations for how best to uphold the integrity of the appointment process to scientific advisory positions in the federal government.[7] And many of the sweeping changes called for by the U.S. Senate Intelligence Committee and the so-called 9/11 Commission in order to better coordinate the nation's intelligence-gathering apparatus similarly speak to the problems of letting preconceived views override technical evidence.[8]

One notable legislative effort has tackled the issue of scientific integrity directly. In February 2005, Henry Waxman (D-CA), the ranking minority member of the House Government Reform Committee, and Bart Gordon (D-TN), the ranking minority member on the House Science Committee, introduced a bill called the "Restore Scientific Integrity to Federal Research and Policy Making Act." Senator Richard Durbin (D-IL) introduced a similar bill (S 1358) in the Senate.[9] Speaking in favor of the legislation, Senate minority leader Harry Reid (D-NV) noted that "President Bush and Washington Republicans have a simple motto. It's partisanship." The Bush administration, Reid said, is partisan even "about scientific facts." But, Reid added, given the administration's many documented abuses, a growing number of legislators like him believe it is time for reform. As he put it: "We believe partisanship should never trump science."[10]

As it turns out, Reid's exhortation may be starting to win the day. Several of the key provisions of the scientific integrity bill managed to pass in the Republican-dominated House and Senate, attached as amendments to an appropriations package for the Department of Health and Human Services (HHS). The provisions, signed into law by President Bush in December 2005, prohibit the deliberate dissemination of false or misleading scientific information at any of the agencies under the purview of HHS (including the Centers for Disease Control and Prevention, the Food and Drug Administration, and the National Institutes of Health, among others). The bill also explicitly forbids administration officials at HHS agencies to question nominees to scientific advisory panels about their political affiliations or voting history.[11]

For those concerned with the issue of restoring integrity to the federal government's handling of scientific and technical information, the provisions represent an important victory. But even the initiatives' staunchest proponents concede that integrity is difficult to legislate. The fact is, in most of the cases reviewed in this book, existing laws or guidelines already stipulate appropriate government procedure; the Bush administration has just chosen to ignore or subvert these provisions. For instance, as reviewed in chapter 8, the Federal Advisory Committee Act of 1972 specifically requires the "fair and balanced" membership of federal advisory committees.[12] When the Bush administration empanels ideologues or vets nominees with political litmus tests, it simply flouts this provision.

Lewis Branscomb, a Harvard University physicist who directed the National Bureau of Standards in the Nixon administration, made a similar observation nearly a decade ago when he reviewed the organizational structures through which presidential advice is given: "No institutional mechanism for advising a President can overcome the President's disinterest; nor will any President desirous of independent advice on a scientific matter have difficulty satisfying his need."[13]

The point is, of course, that integrity in governmental processes requires not only having the right laws and guidelines but establishing a climate in which partisan politics stops at the doorstep of fair-minded scientific and technical assessment. The federal policymaking process ultimately relies upon a complex network of relationships that requires a fine balance of trust and skepticism. For this system to operate effectively, participants must have confidence that government information is accurate and that federal officials are permitted to "put all their data on the table." Only then can policymakers weigh the frequently difficult trade-offs involved in pressing policy issues.

Given the highly polarized and partisan climate in the federal government today, restoring a climate of trust will not be easy. The legislative and bureaucratic efforts above represent an important start toward this end. But the case studies collected here also suggest some additional approaches. As we have seen, the Bush administration has tended to use a recurring set of politically motivated strategies in dealing with scientific and technical information. In particular, it is helpful to look at three overarching Bush administration tactics: tight control of the flow of government information; evasion of accountability; and exploitation of technical and bureaucratic barriers.

Let's briefly consider each of these strategies.

CONTROLLING INFORMATION

As the case studies presented in this book have shown, the Bush administration has been surprisingly successful at censoring and manipulating the work of scientists at federal agencies throughout the government by vesting unprecedented power in a small cadre of loyalists at the White House and requiring that work at federal agencies be funneled through and approved by these officials. As detailed in chapter 2, this strategy has been successfully employed to suppress and distort government information about global warming that conflicts with the Bush administration's preferred strategy of dissembling and inaction on this issue.

In addition, as we have seen, the Bush administration has repeatedly exerted control over government information by suppressing dissenting analyses that have surfaced within the federal government. Usually this has been accomplished through the actions of hand-selected appointees in crucial decision-making positions at the agencies in question. To name just two examples, Jeffrey Holmstead suppressed studies on the effects of mercury at the Environmental Protection Agency, and Stephen Griles suppressed the listing of alternatives in the government's environmental impact statement on mountaintop coal mining at the Department of the Interior.

The Bush administration's control of information throughout the federal government is greatly aided by the dramatic increase in secrecy it has imposed compared to previous presidencies. From the start, the Bush administration created one of the least transparent federal government systems in memory, as exemplified by Vice President Cheney's energy task force, for which the administration claimed executive privilege to prevent public access to even a listing of participants invited to its closed-door meetings. This initial penchant for secrecy was dramatically expanded in the aftermath of the terrorist attacks of September 11, 2001, and has continued to grow rapidly. Some 15.6 million documents were classified by the federal government in 2005, nearly double the number classified at the start of the Bush administration in 2001. At the current rate, according to a recent report, Bush administration officials are classifying as secret roughly 125 documents every minute.[14]

While obviously necessary to protect bona fide matters of national security, widespread secrecy and the uniformly tight control of information in the federal government make it too easy for government officials to lie or withhold the truth and for policies to be based upon insufficient or distorted information and analysis. The record of the Bush administration suggests that excessive secrecy and tight control of information in the federal government have contributed to suboptimal policy outcomes, the stovepiping of information, and the demoralization of governmental staff and advisers.

A remedy, then, is to ensure "high walls" to protect a limited number of vital security matters while fostering initiatives that increase transparency and openness throughout the federal government. The case of the Bush administration shows the price that is paid when decentralized, independent, and autonomous sources of information within the government are lost or suppressed. It also reveals the importance of creating a climate that rewards well-considered dissenting views and analyses as necessary for achieving better policy outcomes. The experience of the Bush administration, in other words, illustrates clearly that difficult policy problems need plentiful sources of high-quality, independent data as well as open, constructive debate and dialogue.

EVADING ACCOUNTABILITY

In addition to exerting a tight and centralized control of information, the Bush administration has systematically sought to bypass and evade many of the checks and balances built into federal procedures to keep the government accountable. In this regard, of course, the administration has been greatly aided by the Republican control of Congress and the extremely partisan climate that currently pervades Washington, DC.

Historically, within the U.S. federal government, the two-party system has helped reinforce the system of checks and balances to ensure that information, technical and otherwise, has been handled with integrity. Similarly, the federal government's network of scientific advisory panels was historically designed to encourage input from a diverse array of scientific advisers and stakeholders. Such mechanisms for accountability cannot operate effectively, though, when one party thoroughly shuts out the other from the decision-making process and even tries to use partisan politics to screen candidates for the nation's scientific advisory panels. To a remarkable extent, this kind of rank partisanship has characterized the two terms of the Bush administration to date.

Close readers of the footnotes of this book will clearly appreciate the effects of this partisanship, for instance, in the numerous references to the work of the minority staff of the House Committee on Government Reform. Under the auspices of Rep. Henry Waxman, this industrious group has exposed many of the Bush administration's abuses, from deceptive practices on climate change data to the distortion of performance criteria in abstinence-only education.

Despite the solid evidence the committee staff—and others—have brought to light, however, their complaints have too often been ignored. Democratic legislators in Congress have been relegated to levying their critiques in toothless minority reports or even in "minority hearings" unattended by their Republican colleagues. American citizens demand and deserve better. Absent the chance for a meaningful check from the opposition party, however, it has fallen to other sectors such as the courts, the states, and the press to serve as watchdogs to ensure that the government upholds principles of scientific integrity.

On several occasions the U.S. courts have played an important role in upholding scientific integrity. In one court-mediated settlement, as we saw in chapter 6, the biologist Andrew Eller regained his position at the U.S. Fish and Wildlife Service after having been fired by the Bush administration for speaking out on the lack of integrity in the agency's handling of technical information about the protection of endangered panthers in Florida.[15] This kind of case is important because government scientists have no specific legal protection should they seek to resist orders or actions by their superiors that violate the ethical code of science. As it currently stands, the Whistleblower Protection Act offers protection only against such abuses if they result in a violation of laws or create imminent danger to public health and safety.[16] Although resorting to the courts is often costly and slow, it remains an important recourse for scientists and government agency staff members willing to risk coming forward when they witness or are party to the government's mishandling of scientific and technical information.

The states, too, can play an important if reactive role in accountability. For example, several states are now suing the federal government to uphold the New Source Review provisions of the Clean Air Act that the Bush administration has quietly undermined at the federal level.[17] And, as mentioned in chapter 5, eleven states are challenging the Bush administration's new rule on mercury emissions. State legislatures have also played an important role in keeping the federal government accountable to popular opinion by overriding the Bush administration's ideologically motivated ban on funding for embryonic stem cell research. As California has shown, the state role in filling the gap left by the federal ban can be substantial: voters approved a bond measure pledging an extraordinary $3 billion over the next decade toward embryonic stem cell research.[18]

Ultimately, though, when it comes to accountability, nothing can replace the vital and indispensable role played by the press. As the case studies have repeatedly documented, the best way to swiftly restore credibility to the policymaking process is to shine the antiseptic light of public scrutiny. Despite the frequent and often well-deserved critiques that today's press is pliant at best, there is no doubt that it has helped stem some of the worst excesses of the Bush administration's distortion and suppression of scientific and technical information. Most often, the credit goes primarily to government officials who have effectively used the media to leak evidence of the overt manipulation or suppression of scientific data; public scrutiny of this information, in turn, has frequently forced the Bush administration to change course.

This pattern began early in 2001, when Bush administration officials sought to overrule EPA research and recommendations and to promulgate a more lax standard for arsenic contamination in drinking water.[19] Based on years of study by the EPA and a 1999 review by the National Academy of Sciences, the Clinton administration had opted to establish a 10-part-per-billion standard for arsenic in drinking water. But when the Bush administration came in, it sought, in a cavalier contradiction of the scientific evidence, to revert to the old 50-part-per-billion standard. After reports in the press led to a public outcry over the issue, the administration was embarrassed into accepting a standard based on the best available scientific evidence.

A similar kind of public accountability was brought to bear in the 2003 leak of the draft *National Healthcare Disparities Report* from a branch of the Department of Health and Human Services (see chapter 3). And, as we saw in chapter 2, leaks to the press played an indispensable role in bringing to light the Bush administration's distortion and suppression of scientific reports on climate change science. Of course, the federal government shouldn't be in the business of altering or suppressing such reports in the first place. But when such abuses occur and when the opposition party is blocked in its efforts to hold government officials accountable for them, public disclosure of the abuses has afforded at least some measure of public accountability.

When it comes to the integrity of the federal government's handling of scientific and technical information, the need for accountability cannot be overemphasized. The goal, of course, should be to create a climate that encourages scientists and technical experts in the process to speak out and that allows for the meaningful participation of all stakeholders involved. The unfettered collection and dissemination of government data and analysis must be treated as akin to other kinds of basic rights embedded in the American system of justice such as freedom of speech and religion. Indeed, it *is* a vital and specialized kind of free speech.[20]

EXPLOITING BARRIERS

Nothing can alter the fundamental need for public accountability on issues of scientific integrity in policymaking. But it is also important to note how successfully the Bush administration has exploited technical and bureaucratic barriers to this kind of accountability. Many of the issues treated in this book are highly complex and technical; as a result, they present high barriers to public understanding. The public is also often unfamiliar with the work of scientific advisory panels and the details of governmental data collection. Moreover, the public has been subjected to a long list of conflicting reports from scientists and other experts about subjects ranging from the link between environmental factors and disease to the safety of genetically modified crops.

Not only are many of the cases collected in this book highly technical; most also involve arcane bureaucratic rules and guidelines. From the bureaucratic complexity of the government's New Source Review provisions under the Clean Air Act to the rules governing performance criteria for abstinence-only education, our ability to monitor the government's integrity is contingent upon our ability to grasp the scientific and technical details and bureaucratic protocols involved.

As we have seen, in its manipulation of scientific and technical information in the government, the Bush administration has benefited tremendously from hiring so many midlevel bureaucrats straight from lobbying positions in industry.[21] These people tend to be extremely knowledgeable about the bureaucratic and technical issues in their fields. They also tend to be so ideologically motivated in favor of their industries that they are frequently willing to relegate the practice of science to the level of "a public relations tool," in the phrase of Philip E. Clapp, president of the National Environmental Trust.[22] In so doing these Bush appointees have too often drawn cynically from the tobacco industry's strategies to foment uncertainty on scientific topics where little or none actually exists and thereby stymie the government's regulatory efforts. Using the moniker of "sound science," these officials actually demean and politicize the government's information-gathering process.

The danger to the scientific enterprise from this kind of attack is particularly great. As Jeremy Symons, a climate policy expert at the National Wildlife Federation and a former climate policy adviser at EPA, has put it, this kind of politically motivated pseudoscience under the rubric of "sound science" is no different from the "White House directing the secretary of labor to alter unemployment data to paint a rosy economic picture."[23] And yet, the public often fails to recognize what is at stake.

This is why the willingness of U.S. scientists inside and outside of government to speak out about these issues has been so important in turning the debate. Both by training and by inclination, scientists tend to be apolitical and are often reluctant to enter the political fray. Yet, whether by signing a prominent statement about the Bush administration's lack of scientific integrity or through other similar efforts organized by professional societies or other groups, the scientific community has offered an important corrective to the Bush administration's exploitation of technical and bureaucratic barriers in policymaking. Scientists, as knowledgeable and politically independent experts, stand at a crucial vantage point from which to alert the public about government abuses of scientific integrity. Even Bush's science adviser, John Marburger, acknowledged this when the Union of Concerned Scientists issued its initial report, for instance. As Marburger explained in an interview: "It was the scientists' credibility that gave the [UCS] report its weight. And that created a dynamic that was very difficult to ignore."[24]

Despite Marburger's retrospective comments, many in the Bush administration tried to portray the UCS report as nothing more than partisan politics in anticipation of the 2004 presidential election. But they badly misjudged the scientists involved if they thought so many of them would readily allow themselves to be drawn into a partisan debate. The inclusion in these efforts of some well-known Republican scientists and policymakers alone ought to have laid this criticism to rest. As reluctant as they are to be drawn into partisan mudslinging, Republicans and Democrats alike in the scientific community have every self-interested reason to be concerned about scientific integrity in governmental processes. Their input is essential for communicating to the public a full understanding of "best practices" and "scientific excellence"—and of the dangers of misrepresentation—in the government's handling of scientific and technical data.

Yet while scientists play a crucial role in alerting the public to scientific integrity issues, this is no substitute for broader public accountability. The answer can never be to cede control to a technocratic elite, however well intentioned. Scientists possess a great deal of technical mastery but, of course, they have no special right to weigh in disproportionately on policy decisions.

Oddly, the Bush administration seems to make the bad mistake of thinking that scientific analysis dictates policy and so tries to suppress or distort information it doesn't like. Sheila Jasanoff, a professor of science and technology studies at Harvard University, has clearly refuted the fallacy that "the facts" present us with some inevitable and perfect technical solution to policy problems. Rather, as Jasanoff explains:

> In regulatory science, more even than in research science, there can be no perfect, objectively verifiable truth. The most one can hope for is a serviceable truth: a state of knowledge that satisfies the test of scientific acceptability and supports reasoned decision making, but also assures those exposed to risk that their interests have not been sacrificed on the altar of impossible scientific certainty.[25]

The problem of barriers to public understanding is further complicated, however, by the general ignorance of science and technology that has reached grave proportions in the United States. For instance, as noted recently in the *New York Times,* Jon D. Miller, a leading survey researcher on Americans' scientific literacy, claims that only some 20 to 25 percent of Americans are "scientifically savvy and alert." Miller, who has been surveying Americans on behalf of the National Science Foundation and other governmental agencies for the past three decades, presents a worrisome picture. His surveys show, for instance, that fewer than one-third of American adults can identify DNA as a key to hered-ity. Twenty percent of adult Americans, according to Miller, actually be-lieve the sun revolves around the earth, an idea that was refuted in the 1600s.[26] Such data points to a huge and challenging job for science edu-cators. It also goes far toward explaining how government officials can get away with even brazen distortions of scientific fact.

BEYOND PARTISANSHIP

Such dispiriting evidence about Americans' scientific illiteracy is thank-fully counterbalanced by far more heartening survey data. According to a poll conducted for the Union of Concerned Scientists after the group's report was released in 2004, the overwhelming majority of Americans showed a keen appreciation of fairness and transparency in governmen-tal processes. Some 83 percent of U.S. citizens questioned believed it was important for the nation's leaders to gather information and scientific ad-vice from experts, including those they might not agree with. Seventy-nine percent of those surveyed believed that it is unacceptable to subject candidates for scientific advisory committees to political litmus tests. And a similarly overwhelming majority considered it unacceptable for government officials to suppress research results or remove scientific in-formation.[27]

The truth is, despite the Bush administration's manipulation and dis-tortion of scientific and technical information, despite a religious funda-mentalist backlash that is surely intensified by threats of job loss and globalization, despite woeful problems of scientific illiteracy, the Amer-ican public does have an abiding sense of fair play and does seem to sup-port the notion that policies ought to be based upon solid scientific re-search and pragmatic problem solving rather than upon the dictates of ideologically motivated fringe groups and industry lobbyists.

These findings reflect a broader and enduring consensus in the United States that has long served as the bedrock of its democratic society. Whatever Americans' failings to comprehend scientific and technical in-formation, the nation has traditionally upheld fundamental beliefs in pluralism, progress, and pragmatism. While there is some evidence of erosions of these values, they nonetheless remain strong. The pluralist tendencies have traditionally recognized the importance of diverse inputs on policy matters and a healthy tolerance for religious and ethnic differences. Americans' deep-seated belief in technological progress has a long and well-documented history. And finally, the fundamental pragmatism of the American public has historically held that most technical issues, like all other governmental matters, can be best resolved when people come together to tackle them.

In short, the first order of business in combating the abuse of scientific integrity involves a straightforward working premise: to restore a healthy reverence for the facts that good governmental policies must be based upon. The case studies in this book illustrate governmental processes that have gone badly awry. In the Bush administration, when scientific knowledge has been found to be in conflict with its political goals, the administration has broadly and systematically manipulated the decision-making process. Clearly, this strategy is badly misguided. Whatever short-term partisan gains are won come at the cost of the longer-term legitimacy and integrity of the decision-making process.

It is surely true that many issues in science and technology have long been highly politicized. But in the U.S. government the process of gathering scientific and technical information and advising legislators has always retained a healthy modicum of nonpartisanship. The integrity of this process—through which leading experts in a given field provide data, interpretation, and advice to legislators and policymakers—is a vital and indispensable prerequisite to informed political debate.

Some of today's most vital political decisions—from what to do about global warming to what dose of mercury ought to be allowable for children—necessarily rely on scientific assessment and analysis. The numbers we derive about whether the planet is warming or what amount of a toxin makes people sick still leave plenty of room for dispute on the best and most effective policies to adopt. But all parties have a vested interest in trying to get the most accurate and comprehensive information we can upon which to base policy decisions. For the integrity of our democratic system and for the health of our children, we can demand nothing less.

Notes

PREFACE

1. "Restoring Scientific Integrity in Policymaking," February 18, 2004, sign-on letter available at the website of the Union of Concerned Scientists (UCS), www.ucsusa.org. See also the accompanying UCS report, *Scientific Integrity in Policymaking: An Investigation into the Bush Administration's Misuse of Science,* updated version, March 2004.

2. See "Uses and Abuses of Science," editorial, *New York Times,* February 23, 2004; and "The Science Adviser's Rejoinder," editorial, *New York Times,* April 10, 2004.

3. Dana Milbank, "For Bush, Facts Are Malleable," *Washington Post,* October 22, 2002.

4. See, for example, "Majority Believe White House Misleads Public, Poll Shows," *Wall Street Journal Online,* November 23, 2005, reporting on a Harris Poll indicating that some 64 percent of Americans believe the Bush administration "generally misleads the American public on current issues to achieve its own ends"; available at online.wsj.com.

5. U.S. Office of Science and Technology Policy, John H. Marburger III, "Response to the Union of Concerned Scientists'. February 2004 Document," April 2, 2004; available at www.ostp.gov.

6. While no major changes were required in its reports, it should be noted that UCS did correct minor details in an updated report posted on its website in March 2004. This version also has an accompanying note explaining the adjustments; available at www.ucsusa.org.

1. FACTS MATTER

1. Richard C. Lewontin, "Dishonesty in Science," *New York Review of Books,* November 18, 2004; available at www.nybooks.com.

2. Mads Melbye et al., "Induced Abortion and the Risk of Breast Cancer," *New England Journal of Medicine* 336, 2 (January 9, 1997): 81–85.

3. "Summary Report: Early Reproductive Events and Breast Cancer Workshop," National Cancer Institute, March 2003; available at www.cancer.gov.

4. Richard N. Zare, "Science Is Not Just a Matter of Opinion," *San Francisco Chronicle,* April 28, 2005. Zare, a chemist, served as a member of the National Science Board from 1992 to 1998.

5. Author interview with senior government scientist, name withheld upon request, April 2004.

6. Karl Popper, *The Logic of Scientific Discovery* (London: Routledge Classics, 2002), pp. 279–80; published originally as *Logik der Forsching* (Vienna: Verlag von Julius Springer, 1935).

7. Rob Stein, "Internal Dissension Grows as CDC Faces Big Threats to Public Health," *Washington Post,* March 6, 2005.

8. For an interesting discussion of this phenomenon, see Rep. Brian Baird (D-WA), keynote speech at the 2004 Integrity in Science Conference, July 12, 2004, Center for Science in the Public Interest; available at www.cspinet.org.

9. "The Foster Affair," editorial, *New York Times,* July 13, 2004. The story was originally reported by Robert Pear, "Inquiry Confirms Top Medicare Official Threatened Actuary over Cost of Drug Benefits," *New York Times,* July 7, 2004.

10. Comments by Steven Galson at a Food and Drug Administration press conference, May 7, 2004. See related transcript at www.fda.gov.

11. See U.S. Food and Drug Administration, "Transcript of the December 16, 2003, Meeting of the FDA Nonprescription Drugs Advisory Committee in Joint Session with the Advisory Committee for Reproductive Health Drugs," December 16, 2003; available at www.fda.gov.

12. See E. Pianin, "Proposed Mercury Rules Bear Industry Mark," *Washington Post,* January 31, 2004.

13. D. Ferber, "HHS Intervenes in Choice of Study Section Members," *Science* 298, 5597 (November 15, 2002): 1323.

14. A. Zitner, "Advisors Put Under a Microscope," *Los Angeles Times,* December 23, 2002.

15. Author interview with Laura Punnett, an ergonomics expert at the University of Massachusetts, Lowell, January 2004. Punnett was one of those dismissed from the study section of the Advisory Committee on Occupational Safety and Health at NIOSH.

16. This list was inspired by a similar one proposed by Rep. Brian Baird, Integrity in Science Conference.

17. Franklin Foer, "Closing of the Presidential Mind," *The New Republic,* July 5–12, 2004; available at www.tnr.com.

18. Ron Suskind, *The Price of Loyalty: George W. Bush, the White House, and the Education of Paul O'Neill* (New York: Simon and Schuster, 2004), p. 108.

19. Ron Suskind, "Without a Doubt," *New York Times Sunday Magazine*, October 17, 2004.

20. As quoted in N. Thompson, "Science Friction: The Growing—and Dangerous—Divide between Scientists and the GOP," *Washington Monthly*, July/August 2003.

21. Richard Clarke interview with Leslie Stahl, CBS News, March 21, 2004; transcript available at www.cbsnews.com.

22. Richard A. Clarke, *Against All Enemies: Inside America's War on Terror* (New York: Free Press, 2004). See also Fred Kaplan, "Richard Clarke KOs the Bushies," Slate.com, March 24, 2004.

23. For an astute psychological critique of the Bush presidency, see Foer, "Closing." See also Jacob Weisberg, "The Misunderestimated Man," Slate.com, May 7, 2004.

24. As quoted in Suskind, "Without a Doubt."

25. E. K. Ong and S. A. Glantz, "Constructing 'Sound Science' and 'Good Epidemiology': Tobacco, Lawyers, and Public Relations Firms," *American Journal of Public Health* 91, 11 (November 2001): 1749–57.

26. See, respectively, Union of Concerned Scientists and Public Employees for Environmental Responsibility, "U.S. Fish and Wildlife Service Survey Summary," February 2005; Union of Concerned Scientists and Public Employees for Environmental Responsibility, "NOAA Fisheries Survey Summary," June 2005; both available at www.ucsusa.org.

27. Public Employees for Environmental Responsibility, 2003 PEER Survey of EPA Region 8 Employees; available at www.peer.org.

28. As quoted in Carolyn Abraham, "No Faith in Science," *Toronto Globe and Mail*, April 9, 2005.

29. Scott McClellan, responding to the House Minority report "Politics and Science," August 19, 2003.

2. "ICING" THE DATA ON CLIMATE CHANGE

1. Intergovernmental Panel on Climate Change (IPCC), *Third Assessment Report, 2001*, vols. 1–4; available at www.ipcc.ch.

2. For a helpful review of climate change science, see www. pewclimate.org. The IPCC projection for average global temperature increase in the twenty-first century is 2.5–10.4 degrees Fahrenheit, based upon multiple climate models and multiple assumptions regarding future greenhouse gas emissions. Regional warming may be greater or less than the global average. For example, temperature increases in the United States are projected to be approximately 30 percent higher than the global average, and the Arctic is likely to experience the greatest warming.

3. See for instance, IPCC, *Third Assessment, 2001*, vol. 2.

4. Naomi Oreskes, "The Scientific Consensus on Climate Change," *Science* 306 (December 3, 2004): 1686.

5. For example, see Shankar Vedantam, "Kyoto Treaty Takes Effect Today: Impact on Global Warming May Be Largely Symbolic," *Washington Post,* February 16, 2005.

6. White House, Office of the Press Secretary, "President Bush Discusses Global Climate Change," June 11, 2001; available at www.whitehouse.gov.

7. Radio interview with Andrew Revkin by Amy Goodman, "Bush's Environment Chief: From the Oil Lobby to the White House to ExxonMobil," *Democracy Now,* June 20, 2005; transcript available at www.democracynow.org.

8. Andrew Revkin, "In Editing Reports, Bush Official Minimized Greenhouse Gas Links," *New York Times,* June 8, 2005.

9. Rick Piltz, resignation memo addressed to U.S. Climate Change Science Program agency principals, June 1, 2005; available on the website of *Environmental Science and Technology* journal at http://pubs.acs.org.

10. Ibid.

11. Revkin interview.

12. Piltz resignation memo.

13. Andrew Revkin, "Former Bush Aide Who Edited Reports Is Hired by Exxon," *New York Times,* June 15, 2005.

14. Ibid. See also, "Former Oil Lobbyist Employed by White House Leaves to Join ExxonMobil," press announcement from the Natural Resources Defense Council, June 15, 2005; available at www.nrdc.org.

15. As quoted in Julian Borger, "Ex-Oil Lobbyist Watered Down US Climate Research," *The Guardian* (UK), June 9, 2005.

16. White House, President's Statement on Climate Change, July 13, 2001; available at www.whitehouse.gov.

17. IPCC, *Third Assessment, 2001.*

18. The White House letter, dated May 11, 2001, was signed by John M. Bridgeland, deputy assistant to the president for domestic policy, and Gary Edson, deputy assistant to the president for international economic affairs; text available at the website of the National Academies Press, www.nap.edu/books.

19. As noted in Piltz resignation letter.

20. National Academy of Sciences, Commission on Geosciences, Environment and Resources, *Climate Change Science: An Analysis of Some Key Questions,* 2001; available at www.nap.edu/books.

21. P. Dobriansky, "Only New Technology Can Halt Climate Change," *Financial Times,* December 1, 2003.

22. U.S. Department of State, "U.S. Climate Action Report," May 2002; available at the website of the Environmental Protection Agency, www.epa.gov.

23. K. Q. Seelye, "President Distances Himself from Global Warming Report," *New York Times,* June 5, 2002.

24. Jeremy Symons, "How Bush and Co. Obscure the Science," *Washington Post,* July 12, 2003.

25. A. C. Revkin and K. Q. Seelye, "Report by EPA Leaves Out Data on Climate Change," *New York Times,* June 19, 2003. See U.S. Environmental Protection Agency, *Report on the Environment,* June 23, 2003; available at www.epa.gov. The discredited report is W. Soon and S. Baliunas, "Proxy Climatic and Environmental Changes of the Past 1000 Years," *Climate Research* 23, 2 (2003): 89–110. The study that discredited it is Michael Mann et al., "On Past Temperatures and Anomalous Late 20th-Century Warmth," *Eos* 84, 27 (2003): 256–57.

26. EPA internal memo, April 29, 2003; available as an appendix to Union of Concerned Scientists, *Scientific Integrity in Policy Making: Investigation of the Bush Administration's Abuse of Science,* March 2004; available at www.ucsusa.org.

27. Ibid.

28. As quoted in an interview with Christine Todd Whitman, *NOW with Bill Moyers,* transcript, September 19, 2003.

29. Revkin and Seelye, "Report by EPA."

30. Author interviews with current EPA staff members, names withheld on request, January 2004 and March 2004. See also "option paper," in EPA internal memo, April 29, 2003.

31. Data collected from ExxonMobil annual giving reports, available at www.exxonsecrets.org.

32. Paul Harris, "Bush Covers Up Climate Research," *The Observer,* September 21, 2003; available at http://observer.guardian.co.uk.

33. Russell E. Train, "When Politics Trumps Science" (letter to the editor), *New York Times,* June 21, 2003.

34. Author interview with EPA official, name withheld on request, January 2004.

35. Author interview with EPA scientist, name withheld on request, March 2004.

36. Chuck Schoffner, "NASA Expert Says Bush Stifles Evidence on Global Warming," Associated Press, October 26, 2004.

37. Andrew Revkin, "Climate Expert Says NASA Tried to Silence Him," *New York Times,* January 29, 2006. See also "The Politics of Science," editorial, *Washington Post,* February 9, 2006; and Michael King, "NASA Joke Has Aggie Punchline," *Austin Chronicle,* February 17, 2006, available at www.austinchronicle.com.

38. As quoted in Andrew Revkin, "NASA Chief Backs Agency Openness," *New York Times,* February 4, 2006.

39. Juliet Eilperin, "Climate Researchers Feeling Heat from White House," *Washington Post,* April 6, 2006.

40. Author interview with USDA official, name withheld on request, January 2004.

41. Author interview with William Hohenstein, USDA, January 2004.

42. USDA official interview, January 2004.

43. Piltz resignation letter.

44. As quoted in James O. Goldsborough, "The White House War against Science," Copley News Service, October 26, 2004.

45. Chris C. Mooney, "Low-Ball Warming," *The American Prospect Online,* June 20, 2005; available at www.prospect.org.

3. DOCTORING EVIDENCE ABOUT YOUR HEALTH

1. U.S. Department of Health and Human Services, Agency on Health Research Quality (AHRQ), *National Healthcare Disparities Report,* July 2003; available at www.ahrq.gov. As a result of the outcry over the matter, the report available at the website is now the restored original draft; see n. 8 below.

2. U.S. Department of Health and Human Services, "Fact Sheet: Preventing Infant Mortality," March 18, 2002; available at www.hhs.gov/news. See also National Healthcare Disparities Report Fact Sheet; available at www.ahrq.gov.

3. M. Gregg Bloche, "Health Care Disparities: Science, Politics, and Race," *New England Journal of Medicine* 350, 15 (April 8, 2004): 1568–70.

4. See U.S. House of Representatives, Committee on Government Reform, Minority Staff, Special Investigations Division, *Changes to the "National Healthcare Disparities Report": A Case Study in Politics and Science,* January 2004; available at www.reform.house.gov.

5. Letter from Rep. Henry A. Waxman to Secretary of Health and Human Services Tommy G. Thompson, July 8, 2003; available at www.democrats.reform.house.gov.

6. See U.S. House of Representatives, *Changes.*

7. See Institute of Medicine, *Minorities More Likely to Receive Lower-Quality Health Care, Regardless of Income and Insurance Coverage,* March 20, 2002; available at www.iom.edu.

8. The two versions of the AHRQ report can be found on the web. As stated in n. 1 to this chapter, the text of the original draft has been restored on the AHRQ website: www.ahrq.gov; the executive summary of the version officially released by AHRQ in December 2003 is available at www.reform.house.gov.

9. Terry McAuliffe, Chair of the Democratic National Committee, "How Does the Bush Administration Solve Health Problems Faced?" America's Intelligence Wire, January 15, 2004.

10. As quoted in "Washington in Brief," *Washington Post,* February 11, 2004.

11. Dr. Clancy's explanatory letter is available at the AHRQ website; see www .qualitytools.ahrq.gov.

12. Author interview with Karen Migdail, AHRQ spokesperson, April 2004.

13. See www.cdc.gov/nceh/lead/about/about.htm.

14. Information provided by CDC Press Office, December 2003.

15. For evidence of the decline in lead levels in children since the 1970s, see www.cdc.gov/nceh/lead/research/kidsBLL.htm.

16. For example, see Centers for Disease Control and Prevention, *Preventing Lead Poisoning in Young Children: A Statement by the Centers for Disease Control,* Report No. 99–2230 (Atlanta, GA: CDC, U.S. Department of Health and Human Services, 1991).

17. Author interview with Michael Weitzman, November 2003.

18. Author interview with Susan Cummins, December 2003.

19. The nominees recommended by the CDC but overruled by Secretary Thompson's office included Dr. Bruce Lanphear, Sloan Professor of Children's Environmental Health at the University of Cincinnati and a former member of the Lead Poisoning Prevention Task Force in the Monroe County (OH) Health Department; and Dr. Susan Klitzman, associate professor of urban public health at the Hunter College School of Health Sciences and the former head of the New York City Health Department's lead poisoning prevention program. Both have published multiple papers on lead poisoning in peer-reviewed medical literature. The Bush administration nominees to the panel were Doctors William Banner, Kimberly Thompson, Sergio Piomelli, Tracey Lynn, and Joyce Tsuji. Dr. Tsuji ultimately withdrew her nomination. For more on their qualifications and links to the lead industry, see the Office of Representative Edward J. Markey (D-MA), *Turning Lead into Gold: How the Bush Administration Is Poisoning the Lead Advisory Committee at the CDC,* October 8, 2002; available at www.house.gov.

20. Ibid. Dr. Kimberly Thompson, an assistant professor of risk analysis and decision science at the Harvard School of Public Health, has no fewer than twenty-two funders with a financial interest in the deliberations of the CDC panel, and at least two—Atlantic Richfield Corp. and E. I. Dupont de Nemours and Co.—were named as defendants in the Rhode Island case against the lead paint industry. Despite their industry connections, a standard government vetting of Drs. Banner and Thompson found no financial conflict of interest that would legally prohibit them from participating in the new advisory committee. See minutes of the advisory committee meeting, October 15–16, 2002; available at www.cdc.gov.

21. Deposition of Dr. William Banner Jr., June 13, 2002, in *State of Rhode Island v. Lead Industries Association,* C.A. No. 99–5526 (Superior Court of RI, April 2, 2001).

22. Ibid. A review of the medical literature turned up no articles by William Banner, but in his June 2002 deposition Banner does claim to have conducted one study in rats and one lead poisoning survey in Salt Lake City, although no citations are listed for either.

23. Author interview with prominent lead-poisoning medical expert, name withheld on request, December 2003.

24. Author interview (via email) with Michael Weitzman, November 2003.

25. *Turning Lead into Gold.*

26. Author interview with William Pierce, U.S. Department of Health and Human Services Press Office, November 2003.

27. Author interview with David Michaels, October 2003.

28. Michaels interview. See also David Michaels et al., "Advice without Dissent," *Science* 298, 5594 (October 25, 2002): 703.

29. B. Harder, "Antibiotics Fed to Animals Drift in Air," *Science News,* July 5, 2003. The article reports on Zahn's research; available at www.sciencenews.org.

30. Author interview with James Zahn, January 2004. Among requests denied was to present a paper at an international joint meeting of the American Society for Agricultural Engineering and the Fifteenth World Congress of CIGR (Commission Internationale du Genie Rural), Chicago, July 28–31, 2002. See also P. Beeman, "Ag Scientists Feel the Heat," *Des Moines Register,* December 1, 2002; available at www.dmregister.com.

31. Zahn quoted in J. Lee, "Neighbors of Vast Hog Farms Say Foul Air Endangers Their Health," *New York Times,* May 11, 2003.

32. "Lists of Sensitive Issues for ARS Manuscript Review and Approval by National Program Staff—February 2002 (revised)," USDA, February 2002; available at www.ucsusa.org.

33. Zahn interview, January 2004. "USDA Agricultural Research Service Swine Odor and Manure Management Research Unit," USDA; available at www.nsric .ars.usda.gov.

34. Author interview with Alan DiSpirito, March 2004.

35. Zahn interview, January 2004.

36. Jeffrey Sparshott, "U.S. Closes Border to Red Meat, Cattle after Report of Canadian Mad Cow Case," Knight Ridder/Tribune Business News, May 21, 2003.

37. For beef trade statistics, see www.fas.usda.gov/dlp/tradecurrent.html.

38. "Veneman Announces That Import Permit Applications for Certain Ruminant Products from Canada Will Be Accepted," USDA Press Release, August 8, 2003; available at www.usda.gov. A Q&A issued along with the above press release adds the following unequivocal statement: "Before we take action, the Department will ensure that there is a strong scientific justification for doing so. All actions taken by the Department will be based on sound science."

39. Author interview with USDA source, name withheld on request, December 2003.

40. See 1994 USDA Reorganization Act, public law 103-354, October 13, 1994.

41. USDA source interview, December 2003.

42. Steve Mitchell, "Groups Question USDA's Mad Cow Decision," United Press International, August 12, 2003; available at wwworganicconsumers.org.

43. USDA source interview, December 2003.

44. The drugs, according to FDA documents, include bupropion (Wellbutrin), citalopram (Celexa), fluoxetine (Prozac), fluvoxamine (Luvox), mirtazapine (Remeron), nefazodone (Serzone), paroxetine (Paxil), sertraline (Zoloft), and venlafaxine (Effexor). Mosholder urged the agency to discourage doctors from prescribing to children all antidepressants except fluoxetine (Prozac), the only antidepressant that showed no link with suicide in his study. More information is available at www .fda.gov/cder/drug/antidepressants/default.htm.

45. Rob Waters, "Drug Report Barred by FDA: Scientist Links Antidepressants to Suicide in Kids," *San Francisco Chronicle,* February 1, 2004. See also Dan Rather and Sharyl Attkisson, "FDA Altered Findings on Antidepressants," America's Intelligence Wire, March 30, 2004.

46. Gardiner Harris, "FDA Barred Expert's Testimony," *New York Times,* April 16, 2004. See also "Antidepressant-Suicide Link to Be Probed," Associated Press, April 19, 2004.

47. See "Dirty Tricks?" *New Scientist,* December 4, 2004; available at www.new scientist.com. See also "FDA Tried to Discredit Whistleblower over Drug Safety Claims," *Medical Letter on the CDC & FDA,* December 19, 2004; Michael Scherer, "The Side Effects of Truth," *Mother Jones,* May 2005.

48. Testimony of David J. Graham, M.D., M.Ph., before the U.S. Senate Committee on Finance, November 18, 2004; available at www.senate.gov.

49. See Rick Weiss, "HHS Secretary Says Agencies Must Speak with One Voice: Some Fear New Controls on Flow of Information," *Washington Post,* January 14, 2002.

50. Graham, Senate testimony.

4. ABSTAINING FROM THE TRUTH ON ABSTINENCE AND AIDS

1. For a wealth of information, see the Emergency Contraception website at Princeton University, available at ec.princeton.edu/news/index.html. See also "Barr Receives 'Not Approvable' Letter for Over-the-Counter Emergency Contraceptive," press release, Barr Pharmaceuticals, Inc., May 6, 2004; available at www .barrlabs.com.

2. Emergency contraceptives like Plan B, according to the Guttmacher Institute, accounted for this portion of an 11 percent decrease in abortions over this time period. Additional information available at www.guttmacher.org.

3. See U.S. Food and Drug Administration, "Transcript of the December 16, 2003, Meeting of the FDA Nonprescription Drugs Advisory Committee in Joint Session with the Advisory Committee for Reproductive Health Drugs," December 16, 2003; available at www.fda.gov.

4. Comments by Steven Galson at an FDA press conference, May 7, 2004.

5. See Gardiner Harris, "Morning-after-Pill Ruling Defies Norm," *New York Times,* May 8, 2004.

6. As quoted in Judith Graham, " 'Morning After' Pill Restricted by FDA," *Chicago Tribune,* May 7, 2004. See also Vicki Kemper, "FDA: Doctor Must Still OK 'Morning-After' Pill," *Los Angeles Times,* May 7, 2004.

7. Correspondence from Steven Galson, acting director of the FDA Center for Drug Evaluation to Barr Pharmaceuticals, Inc., May 6, 2004; available at www.fda .gov.

8. Author interview with James Trussell, May 2004.

9. See U.S. Food and Drug Administration "Transcript of the December 16, 2003, Meeting."

10. See American Academy of Pediatrics, "Plan B Should Be Approved over the Counter," press release, May 27, 2004; available at www.aap.org.

11. Jeffrey M. Drazen et al., Correspondence: "The FDA, Politics, and Plan B," *New England Journal of Medicine* 350, 15 (June 3, 2004): 1561–26.

12. Trussell interview, May 2004.

13. See K. Tumulty, "Jesus and the FDA," *Time,* October 5, 2002: "Though his resume describes Hager as a University of Kentucky professor, a university official says Hager's appointment is part-time and voluntary and involves working with interns at Lexington's Central Baptist Hospital, not the university itself." By way of comparison, consider the credentials of two nominees proposed by FDA staff for Hager's position: Donald R. Mattison is the former dean of the University of Pittsburgh School of Public Health, and Michael F. Greene is the director of maternal-fetal medicine at Massachusetts General Hospital; as reported by OMBWatch at www.ombwatch.org.

14. As quoted in Chris Mooney, "Christian Science?" *Mother Jones,* September/October 2004.

15. Ayelish McGarvey, "Dr. Hager's Family Values," *The Nation,* May 30, 2005.

16. Marc Kaufman, "Memo May Have Swayed Plan B Ruling," *Washington Post,* May 12, 2005.

17. McGarvey, "Dr. Hager's Family Values."

18. See U.S. Food and Drug Administration, "Transcript of the December 16, 2003 Meeting."

19. Berenson quoted in ibid. See "Facts You Should Know about Teenage Pregnancy," March of Dimes, March 2002; available at www.marchofdimes.com.

20. Cicely Marston et al, "Impact on Contraceptive Practice of Making Emergency Hormonal Contraception Available over the Counter in Great Britain: Repeated Cross Sectional Surveys," *British Medical Journal,* July 11, 2005; available at www.bmj.com.

21. As quoted in Ellen Goodman, "Whose Common Ground?" *Boston Globe,* January 30, 2005.

22. See Marc Kaufman, "FDA Rejects Over-the-Counter 'Plan B,'" *Washington Post,* May 7, 2004.

23. As quoted in Lauran Neergaard, "FDA Rejects OTC Morning-After Pill Sales," Associated Press, May 6, 2004.

24. Steve Galson, FDA press conference, May 7, 2004.

25. See "FDA Aide Quits in Protest of Morning-After Pill Decision," Associated Press, August 31, 2005.

26. As quoted in Rinker Buck, "Plan B Casualties," *Hartford Courant,* October 2, 2005.

27. U.S. Government Accountability Office, "Food and Drug Administration: Decision Process to Deny Initial Applications for Over-the-Counter Marketing of the Emergency Drug Plan B Was Unusual," November 2005; available at www.gao.gov.

28. For a wealth of facts about teen sexuality, see the Alan Guttmacher Institute, *Teen Sex and Pregnancy,* August 1999 and related resources; available at www.guttmacher.org.

29. HIV/AIDS information available from the World Health Organization, HIV/AIDS program; available at www.who.int/hiv/en/. See also U.S. Centers for Dis-

ease Control, Division of HIV/AIDS Prevention, fact sheets and data available at www.cdc.gov/hiv/pubs/facts.htm.

30. U.S. House of Representatives, Committee on Government Reform, Minority Staff, *The Content of Federally Funded Abstinence-Only Education Programs,* prepared for Rep. Henry Waxman, December 2004; available at: www.democrats .reform.house.gov.

31. Ibid. The curriculum noted is called "A. C. Green's Game Plan," prepared by Project Reality, 2001. Other curricula reviewed include "Choosing the Best Life," produced by Choosing the Best, 2003; and "Why kNOw," produced by Why kNOw Abstinence Education, 2004.

32. *Content of Federally Funded Abstinence-Only Education Programs,* citing the "Why kNOw" curriculum, 2004.

33. Ibid., citing the curriculum "Me, My World, My Future," produced by Teen-aid, 1998.

34. Ibid., citing "Me, My World, My Future" Teaching Manual.

35. Ibid., citing the "Why kNOw" curriculum.

36. See Advocates for Youth, "Science or Politics? George W. Bush and the Future of Sexuality Education in the United States," fact sheet, 2004; available at www .advocatesforyouth.org.

37. As quoted in Albert R. Hunt, "Abstinence-Only for Teenagers: A Pipe Dream," *Wall Street Journal,* May 2, 2002.

38. Ibid.

39. Advocates for Youth, "Science or Politics?"

40. A. DiCenso et al., "Interventions to Reduce Unintended Pregnancies among Adolescents: Systematic Review of Randomized Controlled Trials," *British Medical Journal* 324 (June 15, 2002).

41. Author interview with current CDC staff member, name withheld on request, March 2005.

42. Elisa Cramer, "Pledge to Teach Facts, Not Ideology," editorial, *Palm Beach Post,* July 8, 2005.

43. See U.S. House of Representatives, Subcommittee on Health, House Committee on Energy and Commerce, *Welfare Reform: A Review of Abstinence Education and Transitional Medical Assistance, April 23, 2002: Hearing Before the 107th Congress,* 2002, testimony of David W. Kaplan, M.D.; available at energycommerce .house.gov.

44. As cited in Advocates for Youth, "Will Ideology Trump Science in Deciding Public Health Policy?"; fact sheet available at www.advocatesforyouth.org.

45. Author interview with CDC staff member, name withheld on request, November 2003.

46. Author interview with former CDC scientist, name withheld on request, September 2005. Subsequent comments are all from this interview.

47. *Government Performance and Results Act of 1993,* Public Law No. 103–62, 107 Stat. 285; available at www.whitehouse.gov.

48. The former performance measures can be found at *Federal Register* 65:69562–65 (November 17, 2000). The new Bush administration performance measures are detailed in U.S. Department of Health and Human Services, *SPRANS Community-Based Abstinence Education Program, Pre-Application Workshop* (December 2002); available at www.mchb.hrsa.gov.

49. Presentation by Donna Hutton, project officer, Maternal and Child Health Bureau, Program Update and Open Discussion, Onward and Upward! SPRANS Community-Based Abstinence Education Grantee Meeting, November 18–19, 2002. Cited in letter from Rep. Henry A. Waxman to Secretary of Health and Human Services Tommy G. Thompson, July 8, 2003; available at www.democrats.reform .house.gov.

50. Waxman letter, 2003.

51. "Too Much Morality, Too Little Sense—AIDS," *The Economist,* July 30, 2005.

52. U.S. Government Accountability Office, "Global Health: Spending Requirement Presents Challenges for Allocating Prevention Funding under the President's Emergency Plan for AIDS Relief," April 2006; available at www.gao.gov. See also Celia Dugger, "U.S. Focus on Abstinence Weakens AIDS Fight, Agency Finds," *New York Times,* April, 5, 2006.

53. Adam Clymer, "U.S. Revises Sex Information, and a Fight Goes On," *New York Times,* December 27, 2002. A comparison of the two versions of the CDC website pages about condoms can be seen online. The original website, CDC, *Condoms and Their Use in Preventing HIV Infection and Other STDS* (September 1999), is available at www.house.gov/reform; the current CDC fact sheet, *Male Latex Condoms and Sexually Transmitted Diseases* (October 2003), is available at www.cdc.gov.

54. CDC staff member interview, November 2003.

55. Thomas J. Coates, "Science, Not Religion, Must Guide Health Policy," *Baltimore Sun,* September 10, 2004.

56. Author interview with Margaret Scarlett, October 2003.

57. Author interview with former CDC staff member, name withheld on request, March 2004.

58. Rob Stein, "Internal Dissension Grows as CDC Faces Big Threats to Public Health," *Washington Post,* March 6, 2005. See also Susan Okie, "Tensions between CDC, White House; Health Officials Say Low Morale Could Threaten Agency's Ability to Handle Crises," *Washington Post,* July 1, 2002.

59. As quoted in Carolyn Abraham, "No Faith in Science," *Toronto Globe and Mail,* April 9, 2005.

60. Ibid.

5. CLEAR SKIES? HEALTHY FORESTS?

1. As quoted in Felicity Barringer, "The Bush Record: New Priorities in Environment," *New York Times,* September 14, 2004.

2. National Energy Policy, May 16, 2001; available at www.whitehouse.gov.

3. Eric Schaeffer et al., "America's Dirtiest Power Plants: Plugged into the Bush Administration," Environmental Integrity Project and Public Citizen's Congress Watch, May 2004; available at http://environmentalintegrity.org.

4. Abt Associates, "The Particulate-Related Health Benefits of Reducing Power Plant Emissions," October 2000; available at www.abtassociates.com.

5. Schaeffer et al., "America's Dirtiest Power Plants."

6. See Christopher Drew and Richard A. Oppel Jr. "How Industry Won the Battle of Pollution Control at EPA," *New York Times,* March 6, 2004.

7. Schaeffer et al., "America's Dirtiest Power Plants."

8. The EPA website provides an overview of the Clean Air Act and the New Source Review; available at www.epa.gov/region5/defs/html/caa.htm and www.epa.gov/nsr. The full text of the Clean Air Act is available at www.epa.gov/oar/caa/contents.html.

9. Author interview with Bruce Buckheit, March 2004.

10. As quoted in Bruce Barcott, "Up in Smoke: The Bush Administration, the Big Power Companies and the Undoing of 30 Years of Clean-Air Policy," *New York Times Sunday Magazine,* April 4, 2004.

11. Buckheit interview, March 2004. See also Bruce Buckheit testimony in Senate Democratic Policy Committee Hearing, "Clearing the Air: An Oversight Hearing on the Administration's Clean Air Enforcement Program," February 6, 2004; available at http://democrats.senate.gov.

12. Announcement of President Bush's Clear Skies Initiative available at www.whitehouse.gov.

13. Natural Resources Defense Council (NRDC) Press Release, "EPA Proposal Would Exempt Power Plants from Key Clean Air Act Standard," August 31, 2005; available at www.nrdc.org.

14. Ibid.

15. Barcott, "Up in Smoke."

16. Tom Hamburger and Alan C. Miller, "The EPA End Run," *Los Angeles Times,* March 16, 2004. Official Jeffrey Holmstead biography available at www.whitehouse.gov.

17. The bill was introduced as the Clean Air Planning Act of 2003, officially titled "S 843[108], a bill to amend the Clean Air Act to establish a national uniform multiple air pollutant regulatory program for the electric generating sector"; text available at www.govtrack.us.

18. G. Gugliotta and E. Pianin, "Senate Plan Found More Effective, Slightly More Costly Than Bush Proposal," *Washington Post,* July 1, 2003.

19. U.S. Environmental Protection Agency, *Final Report to Congress on Benefits and Costs of the Clean Air Act, 1970 to 1990,* October 1997. See www.epa.gov/oar/sect812. See also data from the American Meteorological Society; available at ametsoc.org/sloan/cleanair/index.html.

20. J. Lee, "Critics Say E.P.A. Won't Analyze Clean Air Proposals Conflicting with President's Policies," *New York Times,* July 14, 2003.

21. As quoted in Barcott, "Up in Smoke."

22. See "EPA Proposes Options for Significantly Reducing Mercury Emissions," December 15, 2003; available at www.epa.gov. See also Mercury MACT Proposed Rule and other source material; available at the website of the National Wildlife Federation, www.nwf.org/news.

23. E. Pianin, "White House, EPA Move to Ease Mercury Rules," *Washington Post*, December 3, 2003.

24. J. J. Fialka, "Mercury Threat to Kids Rising, Unreleased EPA Report Warns," *Wall Street Journal*, February 20, 2003.

25. Environmental Protection Agency, *America's Children and the Environment: Measures of Contaminants, Body Burdens, and Illnesses*, second edition, February 2003; available at www.epa.gov.

26. For a comprehensive overview of the Bush administration's handling of mercury regulation, see Lisa Heinzerling and Rena I. Steinzor, "A Perfect Storm: Mercury and the Bush Administration," *Environmental Law Review* 34 (June 2004): 10297–313; available at www.law.georgetown.edu.

27. See Melanie Marty, chair, Children's Health Protection Advisory Committee, letter to Michael Leavitt, EPA administrator, June 8, 2004; available at http://democrats.senate.gov.

28. Molly Ivins, "Integrity of Science," *Austin-Star Telegram*, March 27, 2005.

29. Tom Hamburger and Alan C. Miller, "Mercury Emissions Rule Geared to Benefit Industry, Staffers Say," *Los Angeles Times*, March 16, 2004.

30. Buckheit interview, March 2004.

31. As quoted in Hamburger and Miller, "Mercury Emissions Rule."

32. Ibid.

33. The Clean Air Mercury Rule was issued in its final form by the EPA on March 15, 2005; available at www.epa.gov.

34. See E. Pianin, "Proposed Mercury Rules Bear Industry Mark," *Washington Post*, January 31, 2004.

35. See "Eleven States Sue over Mercury Trading Plan," Reuters, May 18, 2005. See also Kim Krisberg, "New EPA Rule on Mercury Pollution from Power Plants Draws Criticism," *Nation's Health*, American Public Health Association, May 1, 2005; available at www.apha.org.

36. EPA Inspector General Report, "Additional Analyses of Mercury Emissions Needed before EPA Finalizes Rules for Coal-Fired Electric Utilities," February 3, 2005; available at www.epa.gov. See also "On Mercury Issue, EPA a Sellout," editorial, *Atlanta Journal-Constitution*, February 7, 2005.

37. U.S. Government Accountability Office, "Clean Air Act: Observations on EPA's Cost-Benefit Analysis of Its Mercury Control Options," February 2005; available at www.gao.gov. See also Shankar Vedantam, "EPA Distorted Mercury Analysis, GAO Says," *Washington Post*, March 8, 2005.

38. Buckheit interview and author interviews with two other EPA staff members, names withheld upon request, March 2004.

39. Hamburger and Miller, "Mercury Emissions Rule."

40. For a full review, see Environmental Integrity Project, "Stacking the Deck: How EPA's New Air Toxics Rules Gamble with the Public's Health to Benefit Industry," November 2004; available at www.environmentalintegrity.org.

41. Alan C. Miller and Tom Hamburger, "EPA Relied on Industry for Plywood Plant Pollution Rule," *Los Angeles Times,* May 21, 2004.

42. On the composition of the Bush review team, author interviews with Jay Watson, former regional director of the Wilderness Society, February 2004, and Emily Roberson, California Native Plant Society, October 2003. See also www.cnps.org/federalissues/PDFs/CAScientistLetter.pdf and www.fs.fed.us/r5/snfpa/review/review-report/index.html. On the Sierra Nevada Framework, U.S. Forest Service (USFS), Science Consistency Review Report, *Draft Supplemental Environmental Impact Statement,* Sierra Nevada Forest Plan Amendment, September 2003.

43. U.S. Forest Service, Pacific Southwest Region, press release, "Top Forest Service Official in State Accepts Sierra Nevada Review Recommendation, Starts Environmental Analysis Process," March 18, 2003. Estimates of the timber harvest for the first decade under the revised plan are 448 million board feet; under the original plan it was estimated at 157 million board feet. The difference results from a relaxation of the rules on the diameter of harvestable trees, from 20 inches under the original plan to 30 inches under the proposed revisions.

44. Pacific Southwest Regional Forester Jack Blackwell, as quoted in ibid.

45. Personal communication with two members of the Science Consistency Review Team responsible for reviewing the draft supplemental EIS, names withheld on request, June 2004.

46. U.S. Forest Service, Pacific Southwest Division, *Draft Supplemental Environmental Impact Statement,* Sierra Nevada Forest Plan Amendment, June 2003.

47. USFS, Science Consistency Review Report.

48. See *Bragg v. Robertson,* U.S. District Court, West Virginia, settlement agreement 1998; case history available at www.tlpj.org. It is important to emphasize that the EIS in this case, as noted in the *Federal Register* in February 1999, was explicitly directed to find ways to minimize, to the maximum extent practicable, the environmental harm caused by mountaintop removal and valley fills.

49. See *The National Environmental Protection Act of 1969,* as amended (Pub. L. 91-190, 42 U.S.C. 4321–4347, January 1, 1970, as amended by Pub. L. 94-52, July 3, 1975, Pub. L. 94-83, August 9, 1975, and Pub. L. 97-258, §4(b), September 13, 1982); available at http://ceq.eh.doe.gov.

50. J. Stephen Griles's biographical information is available at www.doi.gov.

51. The documents were released through a series of Freedom of Information Act (FOIA) requests by the nonprofit Trial Lawyers for Public Justice, including documents released as recently as January 2004; available at www.tlpj.org.

52. See Trial Lawyers for Public Justice FOIA documents. See also Elizabeth Shogren, "Federal Coal-Mining Policy Comes under Fire: Fish and Wildlife Service Says the Administration Ignored Its Protection Plan," *Los Angeles Times,* January 7,

2004. Evidence of the adverse environmental impacts can be found in the body of EPA, *Draft Programmatic Environmental Impact Statement (EIS) on Mountaintop Mining,* May 2003; available at www.epa.gov. See also Ken Ward, "Mountaintop Removal Damage Proved: Bush Proposes No Concrete Limits on New Mining Permits," *Charleston Gazette,* May 30, 2003, and related articles available at www .wvgazette.com/static/series/mining/.

53. Author interview with U.S. Fish and Wildlife Service scientist, name withheld on request, May 2004. On the scale of environmental impacts, see National Environmental Protection Act of 1969.

54. Memo from J. Stephen Griles to James L. Connaughton, chairman, Council on Environmental Quality; Marcus Peacock, associate director, Office of Management and Budget, et al., October 5, 2001; available at www.tlpj.org.

55. EPA, *Draft EIS on Mountaintop Mining.* See also Ward, "Mountaintop Removal."

56. According to the draft EIS, the lost acreage will occur in Kentucky (255,583 acres), West Virginia (86,587 acres), Virginia (29,224 acres), and Tennessee (9,154 acres). See also Gerald Winegrad, vice president for policy, American Bird Conservancy, and fifty representatives from environmental organizations, letters to President Bush and John Forren, EPA, January 2, 2004; available at www.ohvec.org.

57. See EPA, *Draft EIS on Mountaintop Mining.*

58. U.S. Fish and Wildlife Service scientist interview, May 2004.

59. Email correspondence circulated internally by Cindy Tibbot, U.S. Fish and Wildlife Service, October 30, 2002; included in Trial Lawyers for Public Justice FOIA request documents.

60. "FWS Comments on 9/20/02 Draft of Chapter IV (Alternatives)," circulated internally by David Densmore, supervisor, Pennsylvania Field Office, U.S. Fish and Wildlife Service, September 30, 2002; included in Trial Lawyers for Public Justice FOIA request documents.

61. Email correspondence circulated by Ray George, EPA region 3, December 30, 2002; included in Trial Lawyers for Public Justice FOIA request documents.

62. Memo from John Forren, EPA region 3, October 4, 2002; included in Trial Lawyers for Public Justice FOIA request documents.

63. Author interview with Jim Hecker, May 2004.

64. See list prepared by the Ohio Valley Environmental Coalition, available at www.ohvec.org/action_alerts/2002/09_28/GrilesMTRMeetings.pdf.

65. Winegrad and others, letter to President Bush.

66. Author interview with Gerald Winegrad, March 2004.

6. WHEN GOOD SCIENCE IS THE ENDANGERED SPECIES

1. See Ed Kilgore, "Rove, the 'System Coach,' " at www.tpmcafe.com.

2. See Defenders of Wildlife, "Sabotaging the Endangered Species Act," December 3, 2003; available at www.defenders.org.

3. B. Mason, "Ecologists Attack Endangered Species Logjam," *Nature* 426, 6927 (December 11, 2003): 562.

4. Testimony of Craig Manson, assistant secretary for Fish and Wildlife and Parks, U.S. Department of the Interior, before the House Resources Committee, regarding H.R. 4840, June 19, 2002. Most recent proposed legislation includes H.R. 1662, "Sound Science for Endangered Species Planning Act of 2003." See also E. Buck, M. L. Corn, and P. Baldwin, "Endangered Species: Difficult Choices," *CRS Issue Brief for Congress*, Congressional Research Service, May 20, 2003.

5. Union of Concerned Scientists and Public Employees for Environmental Responsibility, "U.S. Fish and Wildlife Service Survey Summary," February 2005; available at www.ucsusa.org.

6. Julie Cart, "U.S. Scientists Say They Are Told to Alter Findings: More Than 200 Fish and Wildlife Researchers Cite Cases Where Conclusions Were Reversed to Weaken Protections and Favor Business, a Survey Finds," *Los Angeles Times*, February 10, 2005.

7. Letter from Rep. Henry Waxman and Rep. Nick Rahall to Gale Norton, secretary of the Department of the Interior, February 9, 2005; available at www.democrats.reform.house.gov.

8. Much of the cost analysis included money already spent in association with the ESA listing as well as on critical habitat protection for other listed species that occur in the same habitats identified for the bull trout, as noted in the Fish and Wildlife Service "Draft Economic Analysis of Critical Habitat Proposal for Bull Trout in the Columbia and Klamath River Basins Released for Public Comment," press release, April 5, 2004; see news.fws.gov.

9. See *Friends of the Wild Swan v. U.S. Fish and Wildlife Service*, 945 F. Supp 1388; 81 F. 3d 168; 12 F. Supp. 1121; 910 F. Supp 1500; 966 F. Supp. 1002.

10. FWS, "Draft Economic Analysis of Critical Habitat Proposal for Bull Trout."

11. The censored version of the report as released by FWS is available at pacific.fws.gov/.

12. The Endangered Species Act permits FWS to disregard scientific information in making critical habitat designation decisions under certain circumstances. Sec. 4(b)(2) of the ESA states: "The Secretary shall designate critical habitat, and make revisions therein, . . . on the basis of the best scientific data available and after taking into consideration the economic impact, and any other relevant impact, of specifying any particular area as critical habitat. *The Secretary may exclude any area from critical habitat if he determines that the benefits of such exclusion outweigh the benefits of specifying such area as part of the critical habitat* unless he determines, based on the best scientific and commercial data available, that the failure to designate such area as critical habitat will result in the extinction of the species concerned" (emphasis added).

13. As quoted in Sherry Devlin, "Economic Benefits of Recovery Omitted from Bull Trout Report," *The Missoulian*, April 16, 2005.

14. As quoted in Blaine Harden, "Report Condemned as One-Sided: Government

Cut out Benefits of Saving Threatened Trout," *San Francisco Chronicle,* April 17, 2004.

15. See U.S. Environmental Protection Agency, "Clear Skies Act, 2003, Technical Support Package, Section B: Human Health and Environmental Benefits," February 2003; available at www.epa.gov. See also Harden, "Report Condemned as One-Sided."

16. An April 13, 2004, press release announced that the agency would conduct a five-year review of the bull trout listing (first listed in 1998). While this review process cannot derail the court-dictated decision on critical habitat designations, it could lead to change of classification or de-listing for the species, and puts the process to finalize recovery plans for bull trout populations on hold. See USFWS News Release, 4/13/04; available at http://news.fws.gov.

17. See Public Employees for Environmental Responsibility (PEER), "Fish and Wildlife Director Overrules His Own Scientific Panel; Allows Continued Hunting of Rare Trumpeter Swans," press release, April 13, 2004; available at www.peer.org. The non-peer-reviewed report is James Dubovsky and John Cornely, "Trumpeter Swan Survey of the Rocky Mountain Population, U.S. Breeding Segment, Fall 2002," U.S. Fish and Wildlife Service Migratory Birds and State Programs, Mountain-Prairie Region Lakewood, CO, October 2003; available at www.grandjunctionfishand wildlife.fws.gov. The second report is R. S. Gale et al., "The History, Ecology and Management of the Rocky Mountain Population of Trumpeter Swans," unpublished report, U.S. Fish and Wildlife Service, Montana Cooperative Wildlife Research Unit, Missoula, MT, 1987.

18. On August 25, 2000, the Biodiversity Legal Foundation, Fund for Animals, and others petitioned the USFWS to designate the tristate population a Distinct Population Segment and list it as threatened or endangered.

19. Dubovsky and Cornely, "Trumpeter Swan Survey, 2002."

20. See Gale et al., "History, Ecology and Management of the Rocky Mountain Population"; PEER, "Swan Dive: Trumpeter Swan Restoration Trumped by Politics," 2001; letter (with scientific citations) from Ruth Gale Shea, executive director, Trumpeter Swan Society, to Steve Williams, director, USFWS, March 23, 2003; available at www.trumpeterswansociety.org; PEER Data Quality Act Appeal to USFWS decision of previously submitted Data Quality Act Challenge, August 19, 2003; available at www.peer.org.

21. Author interview with Ruth Gale Shea, May 2004. See the 1987 report, Gale et al., "History, Ecology and Management of the Rocky Mountain Population."

22. See Ruth Shea, correspondence to Steven Williams, director, U.S. Fish and Wildlife Service, March 7, 2003; available at www.trumpeterswansociety.org.

23. See "Complaint of Public Employees for Environmental Responsibility (PEER) Pursuant to the Data Quality Act of 2000," Data Quality Act Challenge to 90-Day Finding Relative to the Distinct Population Segment Status of Tri-state Population of Trumpeter Swans, May 28, 2003; available at www.peer.org.

24. Undated spring 2004 memo to FWS director Steve Williams, from Dan Ashe, Sue Haseltine, and Rick Bennet, appeal panel members, "Regarding the Public Em-

ployees for Environmental Responsibility (PEER) appeal of USFWS pursuant to the Information Quality Act regarding the designation of the tri-state population of trumpeter swans as a distinct population segment"; released June 4, 2004; available at www.peer.org.

25. Steven Williams, correspondence to Eric Wingerter, PEER, March 26, 2004; available at www.peer.org/ForestService/fwswilliams_letter.pdf. In his verdict on the matter Williams states that the agency's dissemination of information, including the Dubovsky-Cornely paper, "met the agency's standard for objectivity" as required under the Data Quality Act.

26. Notably, until the review panel's assessment was released in June 2004 under a Freedom of Information Act request, Williams refused to make public the names of the review panelists or their finding.

27. See, for example, United States Fish and Wildlife Service, "Draft Florida Panther Landscape Conservation Strategy," South Florida Ecosystem Office, Vero Beach, Florida, 2002.

28. See *Andrew J. Eller and Public Employees for Environmental Responsibility v. Department of Interior,* complaint pursuant to the Data Quality Act of 2000, May 4, 2004; available at www.peer.org.

29. Author interview with Andrew Eller, May 2004.

30. Eller-PEER complaint, May 4, 2004.

31. For review panel assessment, see P. Beier et al., "An Analysis of Scientific Literature Related to the Florida Panther, Final Report," Florida Fish and Wildlife Conservation Commission, Tallahassee, Florida, 2003.

32. Eller interview, May 2004.

33. Eller interview, May 2004. See also Eller-PEER complaint, p. 14.

34. Author interview with Jane Comiskey, June 2004.

35. E.g., UCS-PEER, "U.S. Fish and Wildlife Service Survey Summary." In fact, respondents to that survey singled out Manson as a key politicizer of science within the agency. When asked what would be the best strategy to improve scientific integrity at the agency, for instance, one scientist wrote simply: "Reducing or eliminating interference from DOI political appointees (Craig Manson, etc.) and their special assistants (especially Julie MacDonald)."

36. See L. Quaid, "Bush Administration Yanks Missouri River Scientists off Project," Associated Press, November 5, 2003. The detailed National Academy of Sciences report, "The Missouri River Ecosystem: Exploring the Prospects for Recovery" (2002), is available at www.nap.edu.

37. See M. Grunwald, "Washed Away: Bush v. the Missouri River," *The New Republic,* October 27, 2003; available at www.tnr.com.

38. Craig Manson, memo to the director of the U.S. Fish and Wildlife Service, October 29, 2003.

39. Personal communication with Chad Smith, director, Nebraska Field Office of American Rivers, and with a staff scientist at the Fish and Wildlife Service, name withheld on request, March 2004.

40. Grunwald, "Washed Away."

41. U.S. Fish and Wildlife Service, "2003 Amendment to the 2000 Biological Opinion on the Operation of the Missouri River Mainstem Reservoir System, Operation and Maintenance of the Missouri River Bank Stabilization and Navigation Project, and Operation of Kansas River Reservoir System," December 16, 2003; available at www.fws.gov.

42. All Army Corps documents are available at www.nwd-mr.usace.army.mil/rec/index.html.

43. As quoted in A. Griscom, "They Blinded Me with Pseudo Science: The Bush Administration Is Jettisoning Real Scientists in Favor of Yes Men," Salon.com, November 14, 2003.

44. As quoted in Amanda Griscom, "Craig's List: An Interview with Bush's Point Person on Species and Parks," *Grist Magazine,* April 15, 2004; available at www.grist.org.

45. See Kenneth Weiss, "Action to Protect Salmon Urged: Scientists Say Their Advice Was Dropped from a Report to the U.S. Fisheries Service," *Los Angeles Times,* March 26, 2004.

46. Author interview with Robert Paine, April 2004. The panel also included Ransom Myers of Dalhousie University; Russell Lande of UC San Diego; William Murdock of UC Santa Barbara; Frances James of Florida State University; and Simon Levin of Princeton University. For more about the panel, see www.nwfsc.noaa.gov/trt/rsrp.htm.

47. As put forth in "Draft Hatchery Listing Policy," *Federal Register* 69, 107 (June 3, 2004); available at www.nwr.noaa.gov.

48. R. A. Myers et al., "Hatcheries and Endangered Salmon," *Science* 303, 5066 (March 26, 2004): 1980.

49. Author interview with Ransom Myers, April 2004.

50. See "Salmon Recovery Science Review Panel Report" for meeting held July 21–23, 2003, NMFS; available at www.nwfsc.noaa.gov.

51. Official statements from NOAA Fisheries claimed that the new policy was required by the 2001 coho salmon court decision. Although the NOAA interpretation of this court decision led to an across-the-board policy that hatchery fish be considered indistinguishable from wild fish in defining ESUs, other viable interpretations could lead to a policy of excluding all hatchery fish from ESU designation (as recommended by the scientific panel) or that hatcheries be closed or seriously modified to prevent deleterious effects on the protected ESUs; see, e.g., J. Lichatowich, *Salmon without Rivers* (Washington, DC: Island Press, 1999).

52. Timothy Egan, "Shift on Salmon Reignites Fight on Species Law," *New York Times,* May 9, 2004.

53. See, for example, Blaine Harden, "Hatchery Salmon to Count as Wildlife," *Washington Post,* April 29, 2004, and Egan, "Shift on Salmon."

54. Joe Rojas-Burke, "U.S. Backs Protecting Wild Runs of Salmon," *Portland Oregonian,* May 15, 2004.

55. See NOAA Fisheries' Response to the *Alsea Valley Alliance v. Evans,* U.S. District Court Ruling, May 28, 2004; available at www.nwr.noaa.gov.

56. J. Lichatowich, personal communication, June 2004.

57. The original twenty-six retain their listing and one new ESU is added. Proposed ESU Listing Determinations *Federal Register* Notice Language, May 28, 2004; available at www.nwr.noaa.gov.

58. Lichatowich communication, June 2004.

59. See Myers et al., "Hatcheries and Endangered Salmon."

60. As quoted in Weiss, "Action to Protect Salmon Urged."

7. BURYING MORE THAN INTELLIGENCE

1. For detailed biographies of the NNSA Advisory Committee members, see www.nnsa.doe.gov/docs/NNSAAdvisoryCommittee-Bios.pdf.

2. The NNSA did not announce this decision; instead it was reported by George Lobsenz in *Energy Daily,* July 30, 2003, and subsequently reported by Global Security Newswire, "United States I: NNSA Shuts Down Nuclear Weapons Advisory Committee," July 30, 2003; available at www.nti.org, website of the Nuclear Threat Initiative. See also Christine Kucia, "NNSA Folds Advisory Council," *Arms Control Today,* September 2003, available at www.armscontrol.org.

3. As stated in its charter, the National Nuclear Security Administration Advisory Committee (NNSA AC) was established on June 25, 2001, to "provide advice and recommendations on matters of technology, policy, and operations that lie under the authority and responsibility of the Administrator, as set forth in 50 U.S.C. 2402(b)"; available at www.nnsa.doe.gov.

4. As quoted in David Ruppe, "Energy Department Releases Nuclear Policy Critique," *Global Security Newswire,* April 7, 2004; available at www.nti.org.

5. J. Dawson, "Disbanding NNSA Advisory Panel Raises Concerns," *Physics Today,* September 2003; available at www.physicstoday.org.

6. Gabrielle Kohlmeier, "After Long Delay, Energy Department Releases Weapons Advisory Committee Report," *Arms Control Today,* May 2004; available at www.armscontrol.org.

7. NNSA Defense Programs Subcommittee Report, *Science and Technology in the Stockpile Stewardship Program,* October 19, 2001; available at www.thememory hole.org. Also quoted in Kohlmeier, "After Long Delay."

8. Robert Nelson, "Low-Yield Earth-Penetrating Nuclear Weapons," *FAS Public Interest Report* (journal of the Federation of American Scientists) 54, 1 (January–February 2001); available at www.fas.org.

9. Author interview with Dr. Richard Garwin, January 2004.

10. Garwin interview. See also Michael Gordon, "Bush Vows to Speed Up Work on Star Wars: U.S. to Abandon Arms Control Treaty," *New York Times,* April 30, 2001.

11. Deputy Defense Secretary Paul Wolfowitz, testimony before Senate Appro-

priations Committee, Defense Subcommittee, February 27, 2002; available at http:// appropriations.senate.gov. See also Associated Press, "Pentagon Sees Sample Rocket by 2004," *New York Times,* February 27, 2002.

12. Undersecretary of Defense Edward Aldridge, testimony before Senate Armed Services Committee, March 18, 2003; available at www.senate.gov. See also Greg Miller, "US Claims 90% Hit Rate in Missile Plan," *Los Angeles Times,* March 19, 2003.

13. Philip Coyle, "The ABM Ambush," *Washington Post,* July 13, 2001.

14. U.S. Government Accountability Office, *Missile Defense: Knowledge-Based Practices Are Being Adopted, But Risks Remain,* April 2003, GAO-03–441; available at www.gao.gov.

15. Coyle quoted on PBS *News Hour with Jim Lehrer,* "Special Report: Missile Defense," September 21, 2004; transcript available at www.pbs.org. And see, among others, Alex Fryer, "Unproven Missile-Defense Program Continues to Stir Controversy," *Seattle Times,* July 21, 2005.

16. For an overview of the Pentagon's missile defense tests to date, see Victoria Samson, "Flight Test for Ground-Based Midcourse Missile Defense," Center for Defense Information; available at www.cdi.org.

17. See, for example, U.S. Government Accountability Office Report, *Missile Defense: Review of Results and Limitations of an Early National Missile Defense Flight Test,* February 2002; available at www.gao.gov.

18. "Faith-Based Reasoning," editorial, *Scientific American,* June 2001; available at www.sciamdigital.com.

19. See Fryer, "Unproven Missile-Defense Program."

20. See, for instance, Fred Kaplan, "Bush's Latest Missile-Defense Folly," Slate.com, March 12, 2004.

21. Fryer, "Unproven Missile-Defense Program."

22. For an overview of the history and current status of the debate over the U.S. ballistic missile defense program, see Congressional Research Service Report, "Missile Defense: The Current Debate," updated July 19, 2005; available at www.fas.org.

23. For an accessible breakdown of missile defense budget figures, see Union of Concerned Scientists, "Missile Defense Program and Budget Summary"; available at www.ucsusa.org.

24. As quoted in "U.S. Missile Defense Testing Could Resume in Fall," Associated Press, July 11, 2005.

25. Government Accountability Office, *Defense Acquisitions: Missile Defense Agency Fields Initial Capability but Falls Short of Original Goals,* March 2006; available at www.gao.gov. See also Wade Boese, "U.S. Missile Defense Capability a Mystery," *Arms Control Today* 36, 3 (April 6, 2006); available at www.armscontrol.org.

26. As quoted in Michael Sirak, "Ballistic Missile Defence: The End Game," *Jane's Defence Weekly,* September 13, 2004; available at www.janes.com.

27. See letter from U.S. representatives John Tierney and Henry Waxman, U.S. House Committee on Government Reform, to Defense Secretary Donald Rumsfeld,

March 25, 2004, protesting the retroactive classification; available at www.house
.gov/reform.

28. Director of Operational Test and Evaluation (DOT&E) Report, FY04, U.S.
Department of Defense, February 2005; available at www.cdi.org.

29. As of August 2005, Christie's reports were notably missing from the Pentagon's website; see www.dote.osd.mil/. See also Kaplan, "Bush's Latest."

30. As quoted in Fryer, "Unproven Missile-Defense Program."

31. Ibid.

32. See "U.S. Missile Defense System Activation Delayed," *Global Security
Newswire,* December 20, 2004; available at www.nti.org.

33. According to cost estimates compiled by the U.S. Congressional Budget Office, "DOD's contractual costs could total about $192 billion for Iraq, about $58 billion for Afghanistan, and about $20 billion for enhanced security by the end of
FY2005"; see Amy Belasco, CRS Report for Congress, "The Cost of Operations in
Iraq, Afghanistan, and Enhanced Security," updated March 14, 2005; available at
http://fpc.state.gov.

34. Ron Suskind, *The Price of Loyalty: George W. Bush, the White House, and
the Education of Paul O'Neill* (New York: Simon and Schuster, 2004), p. 75.

35. Richard A. Clarke, *Against All Enemies: Inside America's War on Terror* (New
York: Free Press, 2004), pp. 30–32.

36. Matthew Rycroft, "Downing Street Memo," July 23, 2002; available at the
website of the *London Times,* which originally published it, www.timesonline.co.uk.
Also available, with much supporting data and information, at www.downingstreet
memo.com.

37. For an overview, see Juan Cole, "The Lies That Led to War," *Salon*
(salon.com), May 19, 2005.

38. As quoted in Seymour Hersh, "Annals of National Security: The Stovepipe,"
New Yorker, October 27, 2003. Bolton's intimidation of intelligence analysts at the
State Department also came to light in a closed-door House Intelligence Committee
hearing to examine the Bush administration's handling of prewar intelligence about
Iraq. See, for instance, James Risen and Douglas Jehl, "Expert Said to Tell Legislators He Was Pressed to Distort Some Evidence," *New York Times,* June 25, 2003. It
became a topic of heated debate again during confirmation hearings for Bolton's appointment as U.S. ambassador to the United Nations in the spring of 2005.

39. Karen Kwiatkowski, "The New Pentagon Papers," Salon.com, March 10,
2004.

40. See Julian Coman, "Fury over Pentagon Cell That Briefed White House on
Iraq's 'Imaginary' al-Qaeda Links," *London Telegraph,* November 7, 2004; available
at www.telegraph.co.uk. For more on Feith's role, also see Mike Nartker, "Pentagon
Office Skewed Prewar Intelligence to Exaggerate Ties between Iraq, Al-Qaeda, Senator Says," *Global Security Newswire,* October 22, 2004; available at www.nti.org.

41. Kwiatkowski, "The New Pentagon Papers."

42. As quoted in Hersh, "Annals of National Security."

43. U.S. Senate, Select Committee on Intelligence, *Report on the U.S. Intelligence Community's Prewar Intelligence Assessments on Iraq,* July 2004; available at http://intelligence.senate.gov. Presidential Commission on the Intelligence Capabilities of the United States Regarding Weapons of Mass Destruction, *Report to the President of the United States,* March 31, 2005; available at www.wmd.gov. This commission was led by former Virginia senator Charles Robb, a Democrat, and Laurence H. Silbermann, a senior U.S. appellate judge and a Republican appointee, and is cited as Robb-Silbermann, WMD Intelligence Report.

44. See for example, Robb-Silbermann, WMD Intelligence Report, fn. 218, "It is still unclear who forged the documents and why. The Federal Bureau of Investigation is currently investigating those questions. Interview with FBI (Sept. 21, 2004); see also Interview with CIA/DO officials (Sept. 3, 2004). We discuss in the counterpart footnote in our classified report some further factual findings concerning the potential source of the forgeries. This discussion, however, is classified."

45. See for instance, Josh Marshall, "The FBI's Review of WMD Forgeries Looks Like a Scam," *The Hill,* July 28, 2005; available at www.hillnews.com.

46. See Neil Mackay, "Niger and Iraq: The War's Biggest Lie?" *London Sunday Herald,* July 13, 2003; available at www.sundayherald.com.

47. For a complete review of intelligence failures prior to the invasion of Iraq, see Robb-Silbermann, WMD Intelligence Report.

48. Joseph Wilson, "What I Didn't Find in Africa," op-ed piece, *New York Times,* July 6, 2003.

49. Mohamed ElBaradei, U.N. Security Council Presentation, transcript, March 7, 2003; available at www.cnn.com.

50. As quoted in Charles Moore, "Colin Powell 'Very Sore' about Having Made Case for Iraq Invasion Based on Faulty WMD Evidence," *London Daily Telegraph,* February 26, 2005; available at www.telegraph.co.uk.

51. "Former Aide: Powell WMD Speech 'Lowest Point in My Life,'" excerpt from CNN documentary *"Dead Wrong"—Inside an Intelligence Meltdown,* aired August 21, 2005; available at www.cnn.com, posted August 19, 2005.

52. Robb-Silbermann, WMD Intelligence Report, "Nuclear Weapons Finding 4," cited in Summary of Findings; for a more detailed explanation, see chapter 1, pp. 76–79.

53. It is particularly noteworthy that Rice had been briefed about the aluminum tubes and yet persisted in espousing the favored line about their use for uranium enrichment. See "Rice Aware of Intelligence Debate on Iraqi Nuclear Weapons Efforts before Making Claims," *Global Security Newswire,* October 4, 2004; available at www.nti.org. And according to the findings of Robb-Silbermann, WMD Intelligence Report, "The CIA had still not evaluated the authenticity of the documents when it coordinated on the State of the Union address, in which the President noted that the 'British government has learned that Saddam Hussein recently sought significant quantities of uranium from Africa'" (p. 78).

54. David Barstow et al., "The Nuclear Card: The Aluminum Tube Story," *New York Times,* October 3, 2004.

55. Ibid.

56. Ibid.

57. Liz Jackson, "Spinning the Tubes," broadcast on the investigative news show *Four Corners*, Australian Broadcasting Corp., October 27, 2003; transcript available at www.abc.net.au.

58. Author interview with David Albright, January 2004.

59. Walter Pincus, "Analysts behind Iraq Intelligence Were Rewarded," *Washington Post*, May 28, 2005.

8. STACKING THE DECK

1. For these and many other brief profiles of Bush administration appointees, see the Center for American Progress and OMB Watch, *Special Interest Takeover*, May 2004; available at ombwatch.org.

2. For a full accounting, including a listing of members and other pertinent information, see the online database of the Federal Advisory Committee Act at www.faca database.gov.

3. See *Federal Advisory Committee Act of 1972*, 5 U.S.C. Appendix 2, Section 5(b) 2 and 3.

4. Ken Lasaius, White House Press Office, January 23, 2003.

5. Robert Steinbrook, "Science, Politics, and Federal Advisory Committees," *New England Journal of Medicine* 350, 14 (April 1, 2004): 1454–60.

6. This and the statements that follow come from author interviews with Gerald T. Keusch, May 2004 and April 2005.

7. Confirmed by Yvonne Maddox's current office at the National Institute of Child Health and Human Development at the National Institutes of Health, June 2004.

8. Keusch interview, April 2005.

9. See D. Ferber, "HHS Intervenes in Choice of Study Section Members," *Science* 298, 5597 (November 15, 2002): 1323; and A. Zitner, "Advisors Put under a Microscope," *Los Angeles Times*, December 23, 2002.

10. Author interview with Laura Punnett, January 2004.

11. Ferber, "HHS Intervenes."

12. Author interview with Manuel Gomez, November 2003.

13. Zitner, "Advisors Put under a Microscope."

14. Author interview with a former NIOSH scientist, name withheld on request, December 2003.

15. Union of Concerned Scientists, *Scientific Integrity in Policymaking: An Investigation into the Bush Administration's Misuse of Science*, February 18, 2004; this and a second "update report," published in March 2004, are available at www.ucsusa.org.

16. Rather than focusing on Miller's scientific qualifications, a White House liaison to the HHS grilled him about his views on abortion, capital punishment, and many other topics. Author interview with William Miller, December 2003. See also

E. Benson, "Political Science: Allegations of Politicization Are Threatening the Credibility of the Federal Government's Scientific Advisory Committees," *Monitor on Psychology: Journal of the American Psychological Association* 34, 3 (March 2003); available at www.apa.org. See also Ken Silverstein, "Bush's New Political Science," *Mother Jones,* November–December 2002.

17. See Office of Science and Technology Policy, "Statement of the Honorable John H. Marburger, III on Scientific Integrity in the Bush Administration," April 2, 2004; available at www.ostp.gov.

18. Author correspondence with Sharon Smith, March 2004; details corroborated with Dr. Smith's office staff during her research trip in the Arctic, June 2004. For quotes, see also John Mangels, "Group Blasts Political Quizzing of U.S. Science-Panel Nominees," *Cleveland Plain Dealer,* November 21, 2004.

19. See Office of Federal Advisory Committee Policy, *Directory of NIH Federal Advisory Committees Functions and Members;* available at www1.od.nih.gov.

20. Author interview with Richard Myers, March 2004.

21. Author interviews with two members of Collins's policy staff, National Human Genome Research Institute, March 2004.

22. Author interview with George Weinstock, March 2004.

23. Author interview with Claire Sterk, March 2004.

24. As quoted in Zitner, "Advisors Put under a Microscope."

25. National Academy of Sciences, Committee on Science, Engineering, and Public Policy, *Science and Technology in the National Interest: Ensuring the Best Presidential and Federal Advisory Committee Science and Technology Appointments* (Washington, DC: National Academy Press, 2005); available at www.nap.edu.

26. W. E. Howard III, "Advice without Dissent at the DOD," letter, *Science* 298, 5597 (November 15, 2002): 1334–35.

27. Government Accountability Office, *Federal Advisory Committees: Additional Guidance Could Help Agencies Better Ensure Independence and Balance,* April 2004, GAO-04–328; available at www.gao.gov.

28. "Edict Limits U.S. Speakers at Bangkok Conference," *Science* 304, 5670 (April 23, 2004): 499.

29. Tom Hamburger, "Administration Tries to Rein in Scientists: Health and Human Services Department Orders Vetting of Experts on Panels Convened by the U.N.'s Health Agency," *Los Angeles Times,* June 26, 2004.

30. NAS comments available at www.whitehouse.gov.

31. Pharmaceutical Research and Manufacturers of America (PhRMA) comments available at www.whitehouse.gov.

32. Author interview with Anthony Robbins, October 2003.

9. STEM CELLS AND MONKEY TRIALS

1. David Horowitz, "I'm a Uniter, Not a Divider," Salon.com, May 6, 1999.

2. See Union of Concerned Scientists, *Scientific Integrity in Policymaking: An In-*

vestigation into the Bush Administration's Misuse of Science, February, 2004; available at www.ucsusa.org.

3. Author interview with Elizabeth Blackburn, March 2004.

4. As quoted in Paul Elias, "Scientist Lauded after Government Fires Her," Associated Press, March 18, 2004.

5. Elizabeth Blackburn biography available at http://biochemistry.ucsf.edu/ ~blackburn/aboutdrblackburn.html.

6. American Society for Cell Biology, "Cell Biologists Oppose Removal of Top Scientist," press release, March 2, 2004.

7. Elizabeth Blackburn, "Bioethics and the Political Distortion of Biomedical Science," *New England Journal of Medicine* 350, 14 (April 1, 2004): 1379–80. See also "Science and the Bush Administration: Cheating Nature?" *The Economist,* April 7, 2004.

8. Leon Kass, "We Don't Play Politics with Science," op-ed piece, *Washington Post,* March 3, 2004. For an interesting critique of Kass's claims, see also Ronald Bailey, "Leon Kass Learns to Spin," *Reason,* March 3, 2004.

9. See Union of Concerned Scientists, *Scientific Integrity.*

10. Constance Holden, "Researchers Blast U.S. Bioethics Panel Shuffle," *Science* 303, 5663 (March 5, 2004): 1447.

11. Letter to George W. Bush from U.S. senators Tom Daschle and Edward Kennedy and signed by twenty-five others, March 22, 2004.

12. As quoted in Elias, "Scientist Lauded."

13. For a good, nontechnical overview, see Farhad Manjoo, "Everything You Always Wanted to Know about the Stem Cell Debate," Salon.com, June 8, 2005.

14. As explained clearly, along with many other facets of the debate over embryonic stem cell research, in U.S. President's Council on Bioethics, *Monitoring Stem Cell Research,* January 2004; available at www.bioethics.gov.

15. Ibid.

16. Manjoo, "Everything You Always Wanted to Know."

17. See D. I. Hoffman et al., "Cryopreserved Embryos in the United States and Their Availability for Research," *Fertility and Sterility* 79, 5 (May 2003): 1063–69. Study summary available as a RAND Law and Health Research Brief, "How Many Frozen Human Embryos Are Available for Research?" July 2003; available at www.rand.org.

18. White House, "Remarks by the President on Stem Cell Research," August 9, 2001; available at www.whitehouse.gov.

19. Stephen S. Hall, "Bush's Political Science," *New York Times,* June 12, 2003.

20. John Marburger III's nomination to become the director of the Office of Science and Technology Policy was officially sent to the Senate September 21, 2001, and confirmed a month later, on October 26, 2001, according to White House records available at www.whitehouse.gov/news/nominations/749.html.

21. Hall, "Bush's Political Science."

22. As quoted in Chris Mooney, "Cell Block," *American Prospect,* September 1, 2004.

23. Hall, "Bush's Political Science." See also Stephen S. Hall, *Merchants of Immortality: Chasing the Dream of Human Life Extension* (Boston: Houghton Mifflin, 2003).

24. See, for instance, Sheryl Gay Stohlberg, "Scientists Urge Bigger Supply of Stem Cells," *New York Times,* September 11, 2001.

25. Hall, "Bush's Political Science."

26. Ibid. As of February 2004, according to James F. Battey Jr., head of stem cell research at the National Institutes of Health, the "best-case" number of stem cell lines authorized for use by scientists with federal funds now stands at twenty-three.

27. Harris Poll, August 2004, as reported in "Those Favoring Stem Cell Research Increased to a 73 to 11 Percent Majority," PR Newswire, August 18, 2004. In 2001, a Harris Poll had reported that a 3-to-1 majority believed that stem cell research should be allowed. Three years later, this majority supporting embryonic stem cell research has increased to more than 6-to-1.

28. For an interesting review of the issue, see George Q. Daley, "Cloning and Stem Cells—Handicapping the Political and Scientific Debates," *New England Journal of Medicine* 349, 3 (July 17, 2003): 211–12.

29. See, for instance, "Senate Still Poised to Loosen Stem Cell Restrictions," Associated Press, August 22, 2005.

30. U.S. President's Council on Bioethics, *Monitoring Stem Cell Research,* January 2004; available at www.bioethics.gov.

31. See analysis in RAND, "How Many Frozen Human Embryos."

32. See, for instance, Farhad Manjoo, "Thou Shalt Not Make Scientific Progress," Salon.com, March 25, 2004.

33. For a discussion, see Mooney, "Cell Block."

34. U.S. President's Council on Bioethics, *Monitoring Stem Cell Research.*

35. See George Q. Daley, "Missed Opportunities in Embryonic Stem-Cell Research," *New England Journal of Medicine* 351, 7 (August 12, 2004): 627–28.

36. A wealth of information, including Douglas Melton's testimony before the U.S. Senate, is available at www.mcb.harvard.edu/melton/.

37. See Chad Cowan et al., "Nuclear Reprogramming of Somatic Cells after Fusion with Human Embryonic Stem Cells," *Science* 309, 5739 (August 26, 2005): 1369–73.

38. Letter from Elizabeth G. Nabel, M.D., director, National Heart, Lung and Blood Institute, National Institutes of Health, to Senator Arlen Specter, chair, Subcommittee on Labor, Health and Human Services and Education, Senate Committee on Appropriations, April 1, 2005; quoted in "The Administration's Distortion of Stem Cell Science," prepared for the Minority Staff, U.S. House Committee on Government Reform; available at http://democrats.reform.house.gov.

39. As quoted in Ronald Bailey, "Censored Science: Speaking out on Stem Cells," *Reason,* July 2005.

40. Letter from James F. Battey Jr., M.D., Ph.D., director, National Institute on Deafness and Other Communication Disorders, National Institutes of Health, to Sen-

ator Arlen Specter; as noted in "The Administration's Distortion of Stem Cell Science."

41. Both quotes in Bailey, "Censored Science."

42. As quoted in Ron Hutcheson, "Bush Endorses Teaching 'Intelligent Design' Theory in Schools," Knight Ridder newspapers, August 1, 2005. See also Elisabeth Bumiller, "Bush Remarks Roil Debate on Teaching of Evolution, *New York Times,* August 3, 2005.

43. For a wealth of information about creationism and the teaching of evolution, the best resource is the National Center for Science Education, www.ncseweb.org. For a discussion of the Discovery Institute and its connection to the Christian Right, see Chris Mooney, "Research and Destroy," *Washington Monthly,* October 2004.

44. See, for example, Michael J. Behe, *Darwin's Black Box: The Biochemical Challenge to Evolution* (New York: Free Press, 1996).

45. The passage is drawn from Percival Davis and Dean H. Kenyon, *Of Pandas and People* (Dallas, TX: Haughton Publishing, 1993); quoted in Jerry Coyne, "The Case against Intelligent Design: The Faith That Dare Not Speak Its Name," *New Republic,* August 2005; available at www.tnr.com.

46. As quoted in Claudia Wallis, "The Evolution Wars," *Time,* August 15, 2005.

47. *McLean v. Arkansas Board of Education* (1982) 529 F. Supp. 1255, 50 U.S. Law Week 2412; available online at www.talkorigins.org.

48. The so-called Butler Act was passed by the 64th General Assembly of the State of Tennessee, Chap. 27 House Bill No. 185, 1925; available at www.law.umkc.edu.

49. U.S. Supreme Court, *Epperson v. Arkansas,* 393 U.S. 97 (1968). This and many other legal verdicts pertaining to evolution are available at www.talkorigins.org.

50. *Kitzmiller et al. v. Dover Area School District et al* (2005) decision by U.S. District Court, Judge John E. Jones III, Middle District, Pennsylvania; available at www.pamd.uscourts.gov.

51. See "University of Calif. Sued over Creationism," Associated Press, August 27, 2005.

52. As quoted in Charles C. Haynes, "Unintelligent Debate Abounds over Intelligent Design," *Ithaca Journal,* August 25, 2005.

53. For a discussion of this research, see Nicholas Wade, "The Human Family Tree: 10 Adams and 18 Eves," *New York Times,* May 2, 2000.

54. For instance, see Harold Morowitz et al., "Intelligent Design Has No Place in the Science Curriculum," *Chronicle of Higher Education* 52, 2 (September 2, 2005): 136. This article cites the work of Alan Haywood, author of *Creation and Evolution,* who writes, "Darwinists rarely mention the whale because it presents them with one of their most insoluble problems."

55. Coyne, "The Case against Intelligent Design." See also an informative overview of the issue by Daniel C. Dennett, "Show Me the Science," op-ed piece, *New York Times,* August 28, 2005.

56. As quoted in Wallis, "Evolution Wars."

57. Philip Kitcher, *Abusing Science: The Case against Creationism* (Cambridge, MA: MIT Press, 1982), p. 35.

58. See Herbert Spencer, "The Development Hypothesis," originally published anonymously in the British journal *The Leader,* March 20, 1852; available at www .victorianweb.org.

59. "Evangelical Scientists Refute Gravity with New 'Intelligent Falling' Theory," *The Onion,* August 17, 2005; available at www.theonion.com.

60. As quoted in Kenneth Chang, "In Explaining Life's Complexity, Darwinists and Doubters Clash," *New York Times,* August 22, 2005.

10. RESTORING SCIENTIFIC INTEGRITY

1. Author interview with Bruce Buckheit, March 2004.

2. Author interview with Richard Biondi, April 2004.

3. As quoted in Alina Tugend, "EPA Air Wars," *Government Executive,* May 15, 2004; available at www.govexec.com.

4. As quoted in ibid.

5. As quoted in Joel A. Mintz, " 'Treading Water': A Preliminary Assessment of EPA Enforcement during the Bush II Administration," *Environmental Law Reporter* 34 (October 2004): 10933–53.

6. See "F.D.A. Aide Quits in Protest of Morning-After Pill Decision," Associated Press, August 31, 2005.

7. See National Academy of Sciences, Committee on Science, Engineering, and Public Policy, *Science and Technology in the National Interest: Ensuring the Best Presidential and Federal Advisory Committee Science and Technology Appointments* (Washington, DC: National Academy Press, 2005); available at www.nap.edu. See also Government Accountability Office, *Federal Advisory Committees: Additional Guidance Could Help Agencies Better Ensure Independence and Balance,* April 2004, GAO-04-328; available at www.gao.gov.

8. See National Commission on Terrorist Attacks upon the United States, *The 9/11 Commission Report* (Washington, DC: GPO, 2004). A review of the report's recommendations is available at www.gao.gov. See also Commission on the Intelligence Capabilities of the United States Regarding Weapons of Mass Destruction, March 2005; available at www.wmd.gov.

9. The Restore Scientific Integrity to Federal Research and Policymaking Act, H.R. 839 and S. 1358, submitted in the House on February 16, 2005, and in the Senate on June 30, 2005; both available at http://thomas.loc.gov.

10. See press release, Senate Democratic leader Harry Reid, "Democrats Unveil Initiative to Keep Science out of Politics," June 20, 2005; available at http://reid .senate.gov.

11. U.S. Public Law 109-149, sections 519a and 519b, December 30, 2005; available at http://thomas.loc.gov. See also Union of Concerned Scientists, "New Law Re-

stricts Political Interference in Science," press release, January 3, 2006; available at www.ucsusa.org.

12. *The Federal Advisory Committee Act of 1972,* 5 U.S.C.; available at www.usdoj.gov.

13. Lewis Branscomb, "Science and Technology Advice to the U.S.A. Government: Deficiencies and Alternatives," *Science and Public Policy* 20, 2 (April 1993): 67–78.

14. See Scott Shane, "Increase in the Number of Documents Classified by the Government," *New York Times,* July 3, 2005.

15. Author interview with Jeff Ruch, director of Public Employees for Environmental Responsibility, which aided Eller in his legal case, August 2005.

16. See the *Whistleblower Protection Act of 1989,* Public Law No: 101-12. 5 U.S.C. § 2302 (b) (8) and (b) (9); available at http://thomas.loc.gov.

17. See, for instance, press release, Office of New York State Attorney General Eliot Spitzer, "States Sue Federal Government to Protect Clean Air Act," October 27, 2003; available at www.oag.state.ny.us.

18. See Ivan Oransky, "California OKs Stem Cell Measure, *The Scientist,* November 3, 2004. See also Chris Mooney, "Cell Block," *American Prospect,* September 1, 2004.

19. See, for instance, "Democrats Blast Bush over Arsenic Rules," Associated Press, March 31, 2001.

20. In this regard, it is noteworthy that the issue of scientific integrity was taken up by the American Civil Liberties Union in a June 2005 report entitled "Science Under Siege: The Bush Administration's Assault on Academic Freedom and Scientific Inquiry." Documenting cases of secrecy and suppression of information on the part of the Bush administration, the report goes far toward linking issues of the government's handling of scientific and technical information with other basic civil liberties; available at www.aclu.org.

21. For example, see an analysis by the *Denver Post* that counted more than one hundred such appointments. See Anne C. Mulkern, "When Advocates Become Regulators," *Denver Post,* May 23, 2004.

22. As quoted in Eric Pianin, "Moving Target on Policy Battlefield; Increasingly, 'Science' Used by Proponents and Critics to Score a Shot," *Washington Post,* May 2, 2002.

23. As quoted in Andrew C. Revkin and Katharine Q. Seelye, "Report by E.P.A. Leaves out Data on Climate Change," *New York Times,* June 19, 2003.

24. As quoted in Philipp Steger, "Pandora's Box—Bringing Science into Politics: The Debate on Scientific Integrity in U.S. Policymaking," *Bridges,* Publication on Science & Technology Policy, published by the Office of Science and Technology at the Embassy of Austria in Washington, DC, April 14, 2005; available at http://bridges .ostina.org.

25. Sheila Jasanoff, *The Fifth Branch: Science Advisors as Policy Makers* (Cambridge, MA: Harvard University Press, 1990), p. 250.

26. As quoted in Cornelia Dean, "Scientific Savvy? In U.S., Not Much," *New York Times,* August 30, 2005.

27. Union of Concerned Scientists, "Attitudes toward Science and Politics," internal survey conducted for the Integrity of Science Working Group, September 20, 2004, by Greenberg, Quinlan, Rosner Research, Inc.; additional survey information available at www.ucsusa.org. For more survey research on public attitudes on science, see Roper Center, *National Science Foundation Survey of Public Understanding of Science and Technology,* available at www.ropercenter.uconn.edu.

Index

Text:	Sabon
Display:	Akzidenz Grotesk Condensed
Compositor:	Binghamton Valley Composition, LLC
Indexer:	Sharon Sweeney
Printer and binder:	Maple-Vail Manufacturing Group